The Table between Us
Food, Cultures, and the Stories We Share

Written by: Arjun V. Patel

Lexington, Massachusetts, USA

All rights reserved, including the right to reproduce this book or any portions whatsoever.

Copyright © 2025 by Arjun V. Patel

MyOM Foundation

47 Topsail Lane, Mystic, Connecticut 06355 USA

Photography by Patel Family Members

To my brother, who adds charisma and energy to my life,

and

To young chefs, who may be inspired by food, ingredients, and adventure.

A Mysterious Brew

By: Arjun V. Patel

Into the kitchen I go with quiet grace

The pot rests on the stove, a steady base

Light sparks a flame, its warmth begins to rise

Reveals the aroma hidden in front of our eyes

The scent of mint engulfs the air so clear

Hands interfere, the lid now drawing near

But the mixture bubbles while the scent is trapped in steam

The grandfather clock chimes, time to get the cream

Light fades, the flame goes out with a sputter

Also awaiting my fresh cup of tea is a toast topped with butter

Table of Contents

Preface	1
Introduction	3

Breads

Vegetable Garden Focaccia Bread	6
Georgian Khachapuri Egg and Cheese Bread	10
Homemade Indian Rotli	15

Salads

Grape & Farro Salad with Pepitas	20
Chickpea Sumac Harissa Maple Salad	25
Corn and Avocado Salad	31

Mains

Hearty Vegetable Chili	36
Classic Tomato Soup with a Twist	39
Classic Pizza with No Rise Dough and Fresh Tomato Sauce	44
Saffron Linguine	48
Spaghetti Squash with Italian Style Tomato Sauce	52
Lemon Garlic Orzo with Veggies	57

Table of Contents

Paneer Burgers — 61

Potato Shaak — 65

Khichdi — 70

Bites

Peanut Brittle — 75

Chia Energy Bites — 79

Chinese Bhel — 83

Esquites — 87

Overnight Blackberry Cinnamon Oats — 91

Drinks

Mango Lassi — 96

Berry Smoothie — 99

Epilogue — 103

Acknowledgements — 104

About the Author — 106

Preface

When my doctor first uttered the words possible 'failure to thrive,' those words landed like a quiet weight on my family and me. It wasn't just a clinical term because it was actually a deeply personal journey affecting my childhood. As a child, I was at risk of not growing as I should, needing extra care and support just to get enough calories exactly when I needed them, every four hours or so. I don't remember all of the details, but I vividly recall the feeding therapy sessions where food became more than just something to swallow, but rather became somewhat of a discovery.

I learned how a simple squeeze of lime into creamy sour cream could brighten it up enough to awaken my appetite. I tasted bold, exciting flavors, like tangy feta and rich teriyaki sauce, two flavors that sparked my senses and transformed eating from a chore to an adventure. Those moments taught me that food was not just about nourishment, but was really about joy, curiosity, and connection.

Over time, my curiosity grew into a passion. I became a self-taught chef, experimenting in the kitchen and studying the science behind food and the rich histories that surround every ingredient. Understanding the chemistry of cooking in the kitchen and the stories embedded in traditional recipes connected me to food on a deeper level. It transformed meals from routines into fun rituals. In fact, mealtimes became powerful acts of healing and cultural expression.

This book is written from that place of experience and hope that lies deep within me. I share for children and families walking a similar path, especially for those who worry about every bite, who need encouragement, and who want to find meaning in mealtime. I want this to be more than just a collection of recipes. I hope to create a celebration of food's power to heal, to bring people together, and to tell stories that reach across generations.

Eating food is at the heart of who we are, literally, as our body transforms everything we eat to give us fuel to live. Food carries the wisdom of the land and the hands that prepared it, reflecting seasons, cultures, and histories. For thousands of years, people have eaten plant-based, local, and seasonal foods. It is those meals that grounded us in nature's rhythms and in our communities. The anthropology of food reveals how deeply connected we are to what we eat, where it comes from, and the stories it carries.

Take garlic, for example, a humble bulb with a history as rich as its flavor. Revered since ancient times, garlic was prized not only for its bold taste but also for its remarkable medicinal properties. Modern science has identified compounds like allicin, which forms when garlic is crushed or chopped, giving it potent antibacterial, antiviral, and antifungal efshows garlic supports cardiovascular health by helping to reduce blood pressure and cholesterol levels. It also boosts immune function, thanks to its antioxidant properties and ability to stimulate white blood cells. Garlic's healing legacy, recognized by civilizations from the Egyptians to the Greeks, continues today, reminding us that food is a powerful form of medicine rooted in culture, science, and tradition.

Today, we live in a world of endless choices and global flavors. It's thrilling but also overwhelming. Have we lost touch with the roots of our food? Have we been distracted away from rich traditions for fleeting trends on social media? This book invites you to slow down, to savor, and to reconnect with the origins of your meals, whether from the soil to the spice, or from the past to the present.

Through recipes, reflections, and cultural stories, I hope to share a vision of food as both practical nourishment and soulful expression. Even when growth feels slow or uncertain, there is beauty, hope, and joy waiting to be found at the table.

Thank you for joining me on this journey where only The Table between Us awaits food, cultures, and the stories we share.

INTRODUCTION:
Is Eating More Than Satisfying Hunger?

Food is more than fuel. It's how we gather, how we learn, and how we express love, identity, and memory. While it meets our basic biological needs, food also speaks in the language of cultures, rituals, and emotions.

As someone with a personal history in feeding therapy, I've come to see eating not just as an act of nourishment but as a layered experience, one shaped by sensory exploration, habit, trauma, tradition, and healing. For years, I've worked with individuals relearning how to eat: reconnecting to hunger cues, rediscovering textures and flavors, and rebuilding trust with food. And through that work, I've come to appreciate how deeply personal and deeply cultural eating really is.

This book began as a blog where I explored recipes and stories from around the world, looking at the foods we choose to eat (or avoid), and why. It grew from a curiosity: How do different cultures understand eating? How does globalization impact our ancestral foodways? Have we lost something essential in our shift toward convenience, trends, and imported tastes?

Our modern world offers more food choices than ever before, and yet, paradoxically, it often leaves us disconnected from our bodies, our environments, and each other. With foods flown across oceans, available out of season and out of context, I wonder: Are we feeding ourselves sustenance, or just consuming calories to feel satiated?

In this book, I invite you to explore my recipes through both an anthropological and sensory lens. Come visit my kitchen through traditions across cultures, reflect on the wisdom embedded in seasonal and local eating, and reconsider your own relationship with recipes you love. Whether you are a therapist, foodie, cultural scholar, or simply a curious eater, this journey is for anyone who has ever wondered about the meaning behind a meal.

Perhaps, in the quiet rituals of preparing and sharing food, we find a way back to ourselves, to one another, and to something deeper that nourishes beyond the plate.

Breads

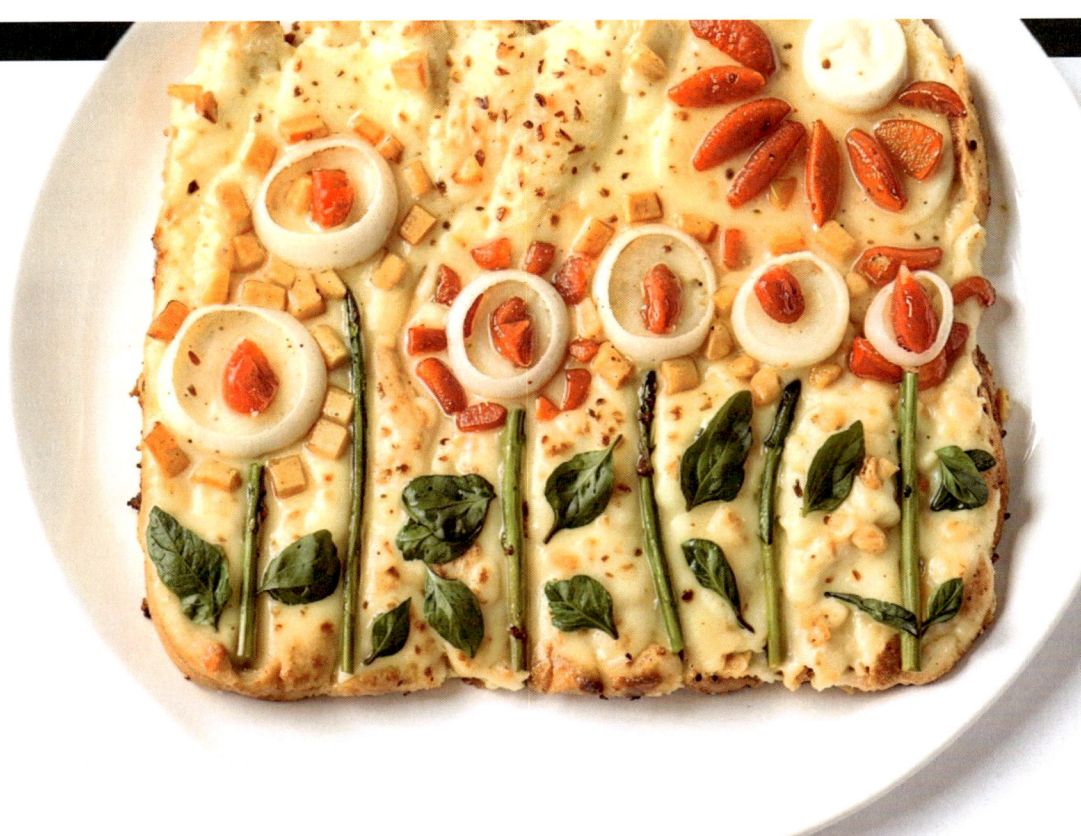

Vegetable Garden Focaccia Bread

WHERE ART MEETS FOOD

Bread, especially yeasted bread, has been a staple in human diets for thousands of years. The practice of baking focaccia in Italy traces its roots to Roman times. By adding vegetables and herbs, we not only celebrate the connection between nature and food but also honor the ancient traditions of culinary artistry. In many cultures, bread is considered a symbol of life and community, something to be shared and enjoyed together.

There's something special about veering off from a general recipe and transforming simple ingredients into a beautiful, edible work of art. This yeasted dough is crucial for the vegetable garden focaccia bread recipe, which is inspired by the colorful produce I find at local farms, which I learned from a local Kids Cooking Green class. This recipe is not only delicious but also taps into the deep cultural roots of bread-making, a practice that has shaped human societies for millennia. Plus, it's a fun, creative way to celebrate the assortment of seasonal veggies!

Ingredients

1 cup warm water (110°F)

1 package active dry yeast (2 ¼ teaspoons)

1 teaspoon sugar

2 ½ cups all-purpose flour

2 tablespoons olive oil

1 teaspoon salt

Colorful seasonal veggies (e.g., peppers, tomatoes, herbs)

Note: Make sure to use active dry yeast, not instant yeast, for this recipe.

Instructions

- **Preheat the oven to 450°F.**
- **Prepare the yeast mixture:**

  In a medium bowl, combine warm water (110°F), yeast, and sugar. Let it rest for 10 minutes until it bubbles and smells yeasty.

- **Mix the dough:**

  Add flour, olive oil, and salt to the yeast mixture. Knead by hand or use a dough hook until smooth and elastic. If using your hands, work until all the flour is incorporated.

- **Shape the dough:**

  On a lightly floured surface, flatten the dough using your palm and shape it into your desired form. Transfer to a pizza pan or baking dish. Use oiled fingers to press and stretch the dough evenly across the surface.

- **Create your veggie garden:**

  Use fresh, colorful veggies and herbs to design a vegetable garden on your dough. Slice peppers, tomatoes, and other vegetables, and arrange them artfully. Press them gently into the dough.

- **Bake:**

  Sprinkle the focaccia with salt and any desired herbs, then bake for 20–25 minutes or until the bottom of the dough is lightly browned.

- **Serve and enjoy:**

  Let the focaccia cool slightly before slicing. Enjoy even more when it's warm!

Pro Tips and Customizations

- If you use your kitchen thermometer, make sure to keep the tip of it within the water and do not touch any part of the container that the water is kept in. This will give you the most accurate reading.

- If you don't have a kitchen thermometer, you can also test the water on your wrist: it should feel slightly warmer than your body temperature.

- Be creative with the veggies based on what's in season or what you may not have tried before—zucchini, eggplant, or even edible flowers could be interesting additions.

- Don't worry about the shapes of the veggies as you are cutting them! You can use your artistic side to create a design on the bread.

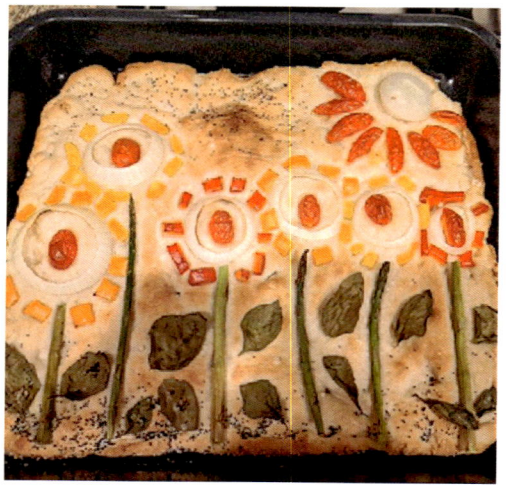

I hope this Vegetable Garden Focaccia Bread inspires you to get creative with your culinary skills! Whether you're a seasoned bread maker or a beginner, this recipe offers a fun, artistic twist on traditional focaccia. Go and get your family involved. You could even set up a cooking competition with friends or family members and show off all of the individual creations!

Georgian Khachapuri Egg and Cheese Bread:

AN EDIBLE BOAT

The Georgian food, Khachapuri, derives from "Khacho," meaning cheese, and "Puri," meaning bread. Khachapuri is one of Georgia's most well-known dishes. But Khachapuri represents more than just sustenance; it carries cultural meaning. According to my classmate and friend, when it is served in houses to guests, it is a symbol of hospitality, friendship, and tradition. Sharing and serving khachapuri is a traditional way to demonstrate hospitality, build community, and express cultural pride.

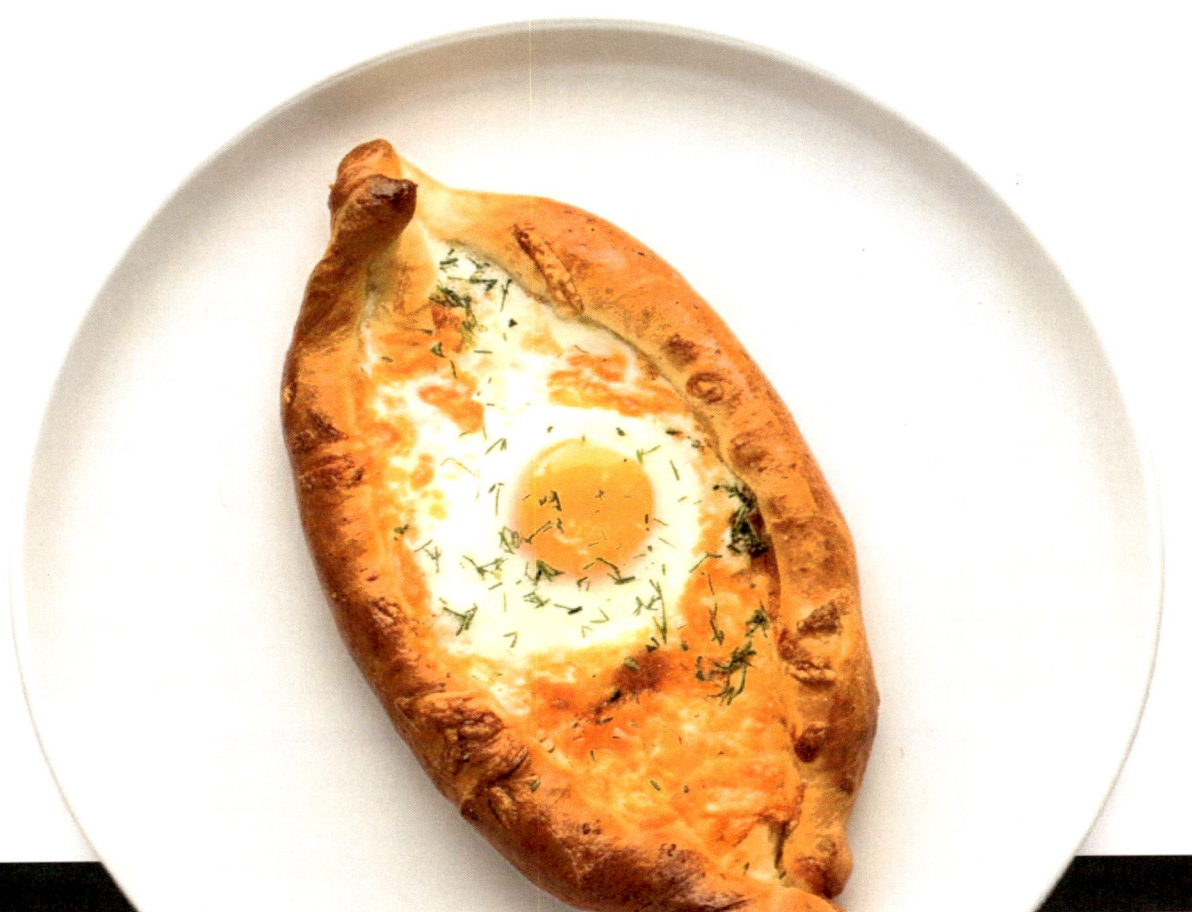

Different regions of Georgia have their own versions of Khachapuri, which reflect the diversity of the local culture and geography. For example:

- Adjaruli Khachapuri (from the region of Adjara) is shaped like a boat and often filled with an egg on top of the cheese. This is the one I make!

- Imeretian Khachapuri (from the Imereti region) is round and filled with a simple cheese mixture.

- Mingrelian Khachapuri is topped with extra cheese, giving it a more decadent twist.

The ingredients used, cheese, flour, and eggs, are linked to the local agricultural practices of Georgia. The geography of Georgia is largely rural and mountainous. The way different regions have adapted the dish to their specific circumstances, like the addition of an egg in Adjaruli Khachapuri, is due to the abundance of eggs in that region. This shows how geography shapes culinary traditions. The regional variation highlights how Khachapuri is both a unifying cultural icon and a reflection of local traditions.

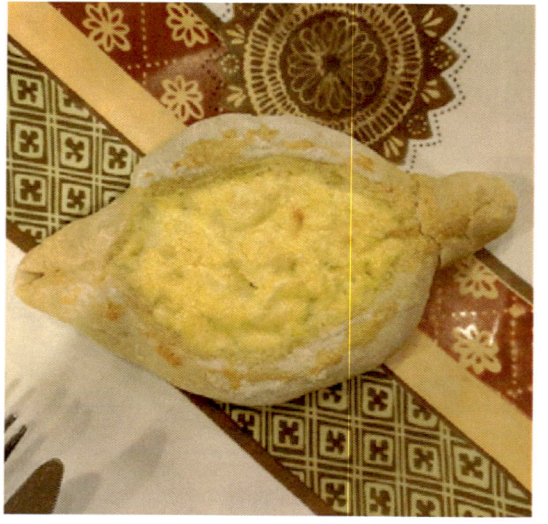

During the pandemic, my classmates shared favorite food recipes with each other so that we could compile them into a memory book and try to stay connected with one another. This Georgian Adjaruli khachapuri egg and cheese bread recipe is inspired by one of the recipes from that class book. This recipe is not only delicious but also taps into the deep cultural roots of ancient Georgia, where it evolved into a gesture of welcome and friendship.

Bread that is best served warm and fresh! It's made individually for each person!

The great thing about this recipe is that you create the serving size based on how you shape the dough for each individual.

Ingredients

DOUGH:	FILLING:
1 cup warm water (110°F)	1 cup mozzarella cheese
1 package active dry yeast (2 ¼ teaspoons)	1 cup feta cheese
1 teaspoon sugar	3 large eggs
2 ½ cups all-purpose flour	
2 tablespoons olive oil	
1 teaspoon salt	

Instructions

- **Prepare the yeast mixture:**
  In a medium bowl, combine warm water (110°F), yeast, and sugar. Let it rest for 10 minutes until it bubbles and smells yeasty.
- **Mix the dough:**
  Add flour, olive oil, and salt to the yeast mixture. Knead by hand or use a dough hook until smooth and elastic. If using your hands, work until all the flour is incorporated.

- **Let the dough rise.**

  Wait for the dough to double in size, or about 2 hours.

  Preheat the oven to 450°F.

- **Shape the dough**

  On a lightly floured surface, flatten the dough using your palm and shape it into your desired boat form. With this amount of dough, usually you can make 3. Transfer to a pizza pan or baking dish.

  Add the cheese into the center of the boat.

  Make an indent with a fork before cracking the egg into the center.

- **Bake for 10-12 minutes.**
- **Second Bake for 3-4 minutes:**
- **Serve and enjoy:**

  Let the bread cool slightly before plating. Enjoy working with warm bread with a fork and knife. Or just take it in your hands and enjoy!

Pro Tips and Customization

- After kneading the dough, let it rest for at least 1 hour to develop the gluten and create a stretchy, airy texture.

- Traditionally, the yolk should be runny, while the white is just barely set. My preference is to cook the egg a bit more. Keep a close eye so you get your desired consistency.

I hope this unique Georgian dish inspires you to get creative with your culinary skills! Khachapuri can be adapted to the preferences of your guests or whatever you have in the fridge. Don't be shy about choosing your own favorite cheese or milk and creating your own version. Invite your friends or family and show off your hospitality, love, and gratitude through this dish!

Homemade Indian Rotli:

SOFT AND PUFFED ROLLED BREAD

Rotli is more than just flatbread; it's a symbol of daily nourishment and community in Indian culture. This traditional bread, made with simple ingredients, reflects the philosophy of using whole, unprocessed foods in everyday meals. In India, rotli-making is a communal activity that brings families together, with each household often developing its own unique technique. Learning to roll and cook rotli is a skill passed down through generations, representing not only culinary heritage but also the warmth and hospitality of Indian culture. Whether served with dal, sabzi (vegetable dishes), or ghee, rotli holds a place in nearly every Indian meal.

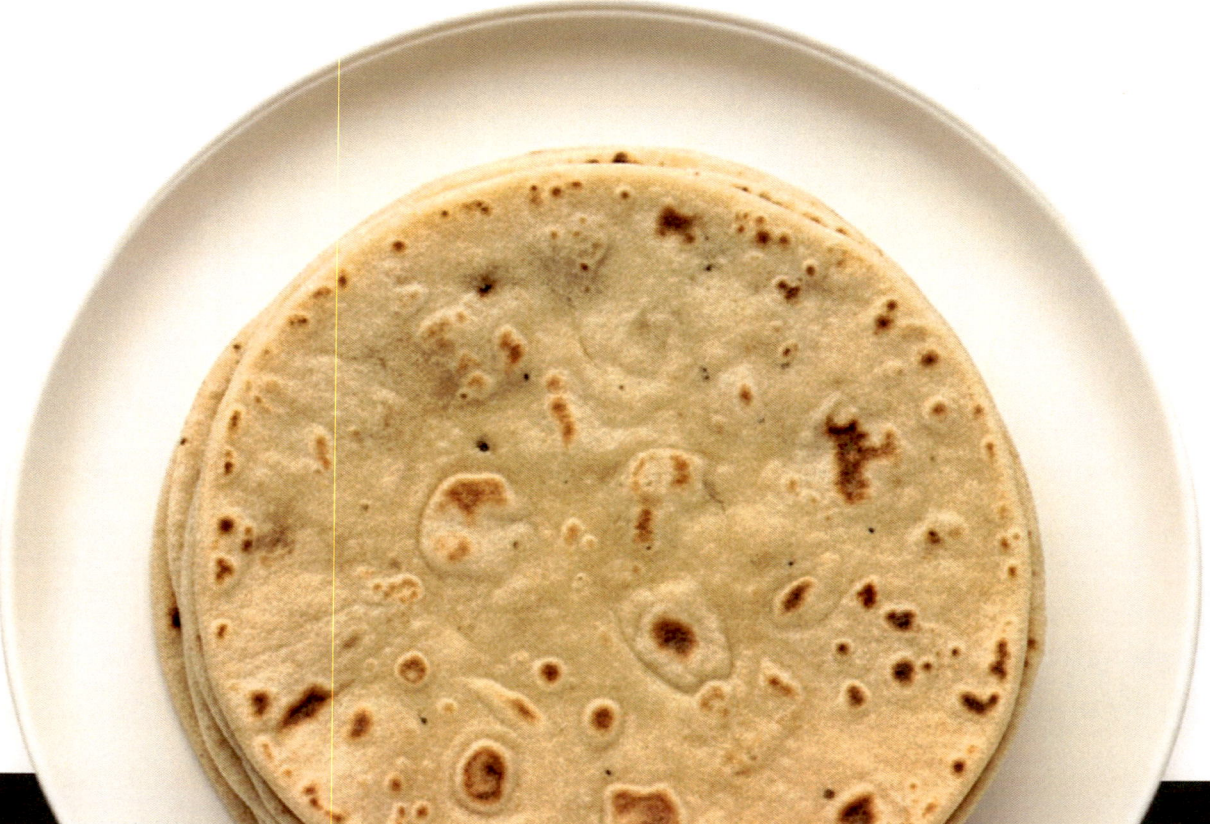

Learning to make rotli, also known as roti, chapatti, or phulka, is a humbling experience as you grapple with the "atta", made from whole wheat flour to create perfectly circular, soft, puffed-up rotli that captures the essence of this beloved bread. Challenge yourself and have some fun too!

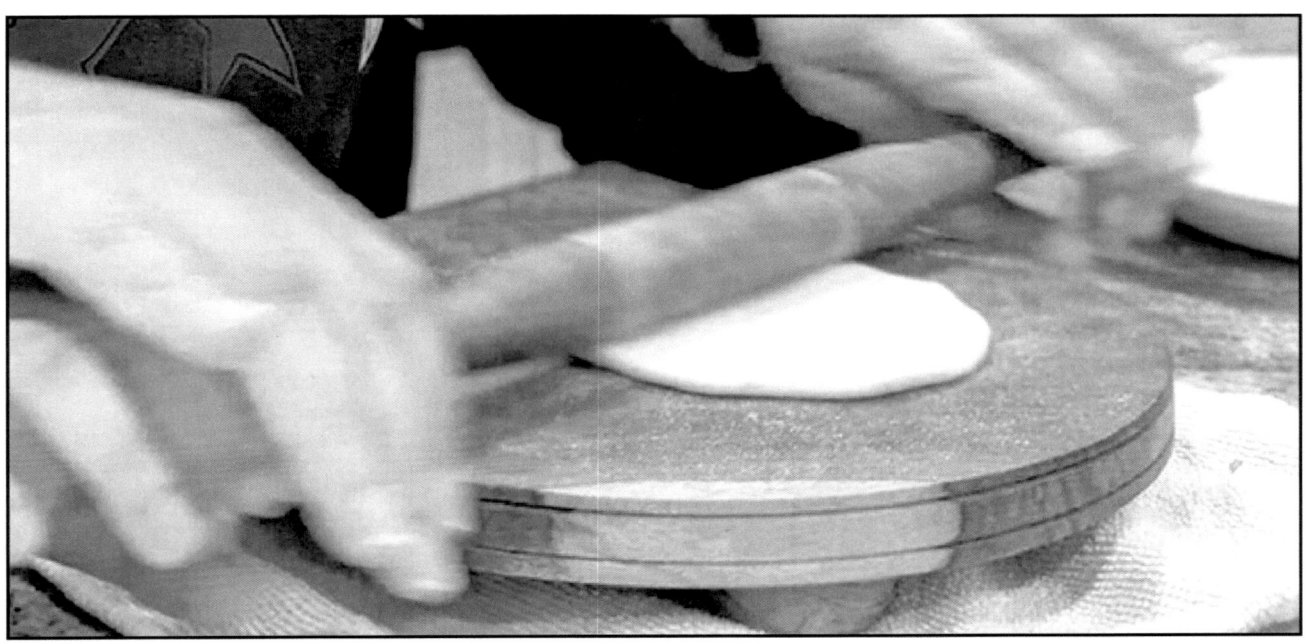

Ingredients

FOR THE DOUGH

2 cups atta (whole wheat flour)

¼ teaspoon salt (optional)

¾ cup + 2 tablespoons lukewarm water (add gradually)

2 teaspoons oil

FOR DUSTING AND ROLLING

⅓ cup atta (whole wheat flour)

OPTIONAL

Ghee or butter, for serving

Instructions

- **To Knead the Dough:**

1. In a large mixing bowl, combine 2 cups of atta and salt. Gradually add lukewarm water, about ¼ cup at a time, mixing with your hands, a spatula, or a wooden spoon.
2. Once the dough starts forming a shaggy consistency, knead it by hand. Use your knuckles, fingers, and palms to work the dough. As it comes together, add the oil and continue kneading until the dough is smooth and pliable, about 4-5 minutes.
3. Cover the dough with a damp cloth and allow it to rest for 15-20 minutes. This resting period helps soften the dough by allowing gluten to develop, making the rotli softer and easier to roll.

- **To Roll the Rotlis:**

1. Divide the dough into 12 equal portions, rolling each portion into a smooth ball. Keep the dough balls covered with a damp cloth.
2. Place the ⅓ cup of flour on a plate for dusting. Take one dough ball, flatten it in your hand, and dip it in the dry flour. Shake off any excess flour.
3. With a rolling pin, roll from the center outwards, rotating the dough ball about 45 degrees between each roll to create an even, round disc. Dust with flour as needed to prevent sticking.
4. Continue until the dough disc is about 8 inches in diameter. Preheat a tawa or skillet over medium-high heat in the meantime.

- **To Cook the Rotli:**

1. Dust off any excess flour from the rolled rotli. Place it flat on the hot tawa. Cook for about 30 seconds, until small bubbles form.
2. Flip the rotli using tongs. Cook the other side until air pockets form, about another 30 seconds. Flip it once more.
3. Using tongs, place the rotli directly over the flame to puff up, rotating for even cooking. If you're using an electric stove, use a flat spatula to press gently on the roti while rotating until it puffs.

4. Remove the rotli from the tawa. For added flavor, brush with ghee or butter while it's still warm.

- **To Serve and Store:**
1. Serve the warm roti immediately, alongside your favorite dishes.
2. Store leftovers in an airtight container or wrapped in aluminum foil to keep them soft. Roti dough can be stored in the fridge for up to 3 days.

Pro Tips and Customizations

- Soft Dough is Key: Ensure the dough is soft and pliable by adjusting water or flour as needed. Let it rest covered for 15-20 minutes to relax the gluten, which makes the rotli soft. Also, try making the dough with milk instead of water!

- Even Rolling Technique: Roll from the center outward, turning the dough frequently to maintain an even thickness, which helps it puff up.

- Hot Tawa or Flame Puffing: A hot tawa is essential for even cooking. Puffing directly over an open flame adds that authentic, pillowy texture.

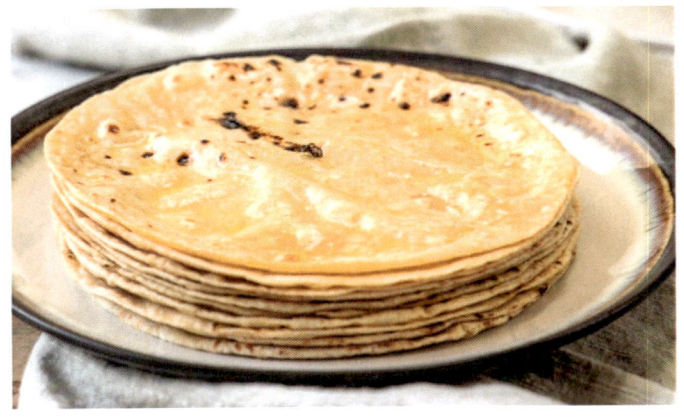

I hope this guide inspires you to make rotli at home and experience the warmth of this timeless flatbread. If you can master this technique, you can impress your friends with puffy, round ball-like breads that soften in your mouth!

Salads

Grape & Farro Salad with Pepitas:

A WHOLESOME BLEND OF ANCIENT GRAINS AND MODERN FLAIR

Farro, a grain with roots in ancient Mesopotamia, has found its way into contemporary kitchens as a versatile and nutritious ingredient. This grape & farro salad with pepitas combines the earthy chew of farro with the natural sweetness of charred grapes, the crunch of roasted pepitas, and the salty tang of cotija cheese. The dish's medley of textures and flavors makes it both a hearty side and a satisfying main course. With its balance of ancient ingredients and modern techniques, this recipe invites you to explore the cultural and historical significance of farro while savoring a dish that's perfect for any occasion.

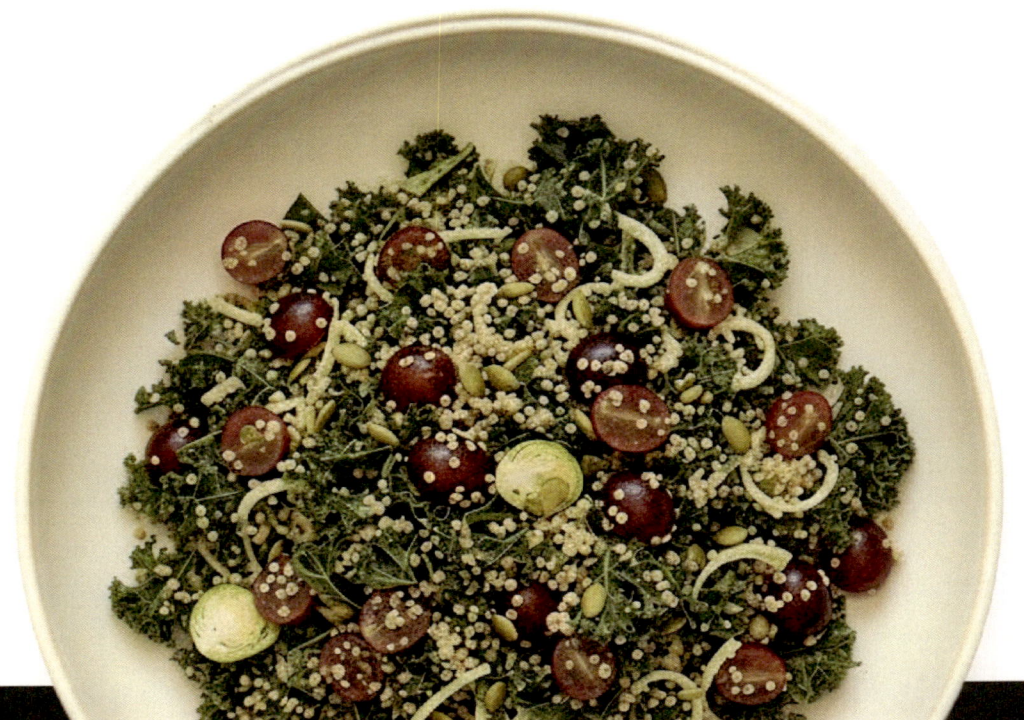

Farro, a grain with roots in ancient Mesopotamia, has found its way into contemporary kitchens as a versatile and nutritious ingredient. This grape & farro salad with pepitas combines the earthy chew of farro with the natural sweetness of charred grapes, the crunch of roasted pepitas, and the salty tang of cotija cheese. The dish's medley of textures and flavors makes it both a hearty side and a satisfying main course. With its balance of ancient ingredients and modern techniques, this recipe invites you to explore the cultural and historical significance of farro while savoring a dish that's perfect for any occasion.

Farro, one of the oldest cultivated grains, has been a dietary staple in the Mediterranean for thousands of years. Its resilience and adaptability made it a favored crop in ancient Rome, where it symbolized abundance and sustenance. Pepitas, or pumpkin seeds, have deep roots in Indigenous Mesoamerican cuisine, where they've been used for centuries in both savory and sweet dishes. This salad embodies a harmonious blend of global culinary traditions, showcasing how diverse cultures influence modern recipes.

Quick Recipe Overview

Dish: Grape & Farro Salad with Pepitas

Cook Time: 15 minutes

Prep Time: 10

Serves: 4 as a side or 2 as a main

Ingredients

FOR THE SALAD:

1 cup pearled farro: An ancient grain, once a staple in Roman diets, known for its nutty flavor.

2 cups water: To cook the farro.

½ lb. red grapes (on the vine): Adds a burst of natural sweetness.

¼ cup roasted salted pepitas: Pumpkin seeds that bring crunch and a hint of salt.

2 oz. cotija cheese: A crumbly Mexican cheese that adds a salty and creamy touch.

¼ (0.75 oz.) pkg chives: For garnish and a mild onion flavor.

FOR THE DRESSING:

2 tbsp. olive oil: Adds richness and ties the ingredients together.

¼ tsp ground cayenne pepper: For a subtle kick of heat.

¼ cup sherry vinegar: Provides a tangy, slightly sweet acidity.

SEASONINGS:

Salt and freshly ground black pepper: To taste.

Instructions

Cook the Farro:

1. In a multi-cooker or electric pressure cooker, combine the farro and 2 cups of water. Seal the lid and bring to high pressure.
2. Cook for 8 minutes under pressure. Allow the pressure to release naturally for 5 minutes, then switch to quick release. Drain any excess liquid and set aside.

Prepare the Grapes:

1. Preheat the grill to medium-high.
2. In a large bowl, combine olive oil, cayenne pepper, salt, and black pepper.
3. Add the grapes, gently tossing to coat while keeping them on the vine.
4. Place the grapes on the grill and cook for 3–4 minutes, or until lightly charred. Transfer to a cutting board and let cool slightly before removing them from the vine.

Assemble the Salad:

1. In the large bowl with the remaining dressing, add the cooked farro, charred grapes, sherry vinegar, and pepitas.
2. Crumble the cotija cheese into the bowl and toss gently to combine.
3. Adjust seasoning with additional salt and pepper, if needed.

Garnish and Serve:

1. Chop the chives and sprinkle them over the salad as a garnish.
2. Serve immediately or at room temperature.

Pro Tips and Customizations

- Make it Vegan: Swap cotija cheese with a plant-based feta alternative or nutritional yeast.

- Try Other Grains: Substitute farro with barley or quinoa for a different texture.

- Experiment with Grapes: Use green grapes or try roasting with a drizzle of honey for added sweetness.

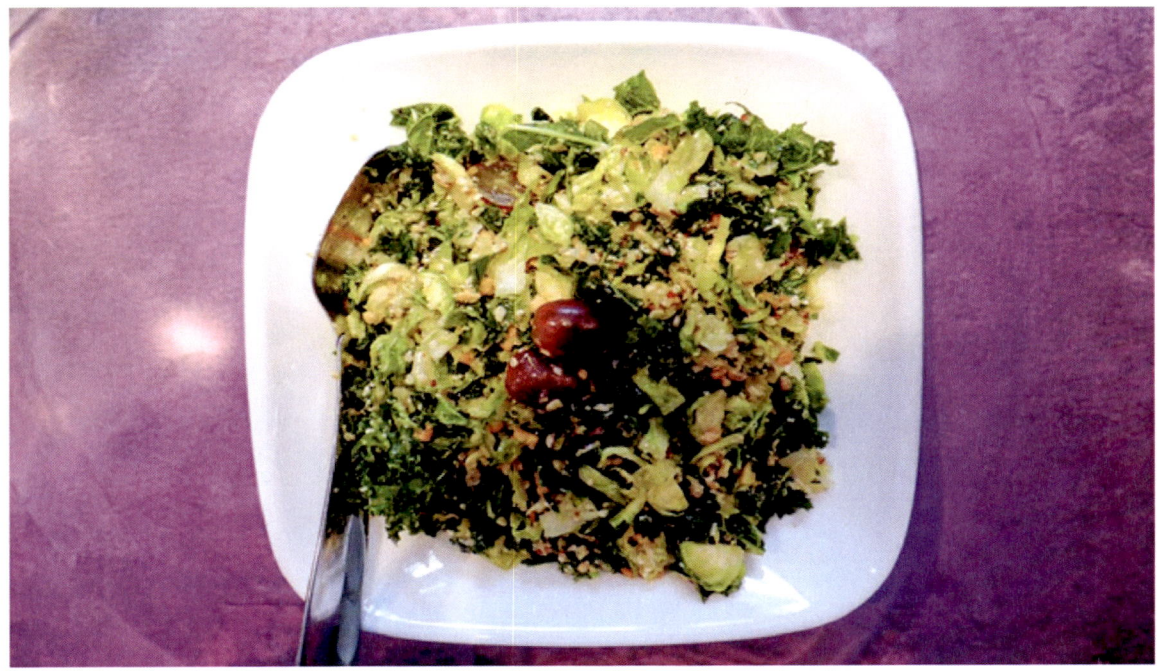

The grape & farro salad with pepitas is more than just a meal; it's a culinary experience that bridges ancient grains with modern techniques. Perfect for gatherings or a quiet dinner at home, this salad is as delightful to eat as it is to prepare. Enjoy exploring the flavors of history on your plate!

Chickpea Sumac Harissa Maple Salad:

A FUSION OF BOLD FLAVORS AND RICH TRADITIONS

Salads are often perceived as light and simple, but this chickpea sumac harissa maple salad shatters that notion with its vibrant mix of bold flavors and nourishing ingredients. This recipe comes from my cousin's cooking class, where our family comes together with culinary creativity and cultural appreciation. The use of sumac and harissa ties this salad to Middle Eastern and North African cuisines, while maple syrup offers a distinctly North American touch. Together, they create a dish that's both complex and comforting. Join in exploring the cultural significance behind these ingredients and dive into a recipe that is as satisfying as it is colorful.

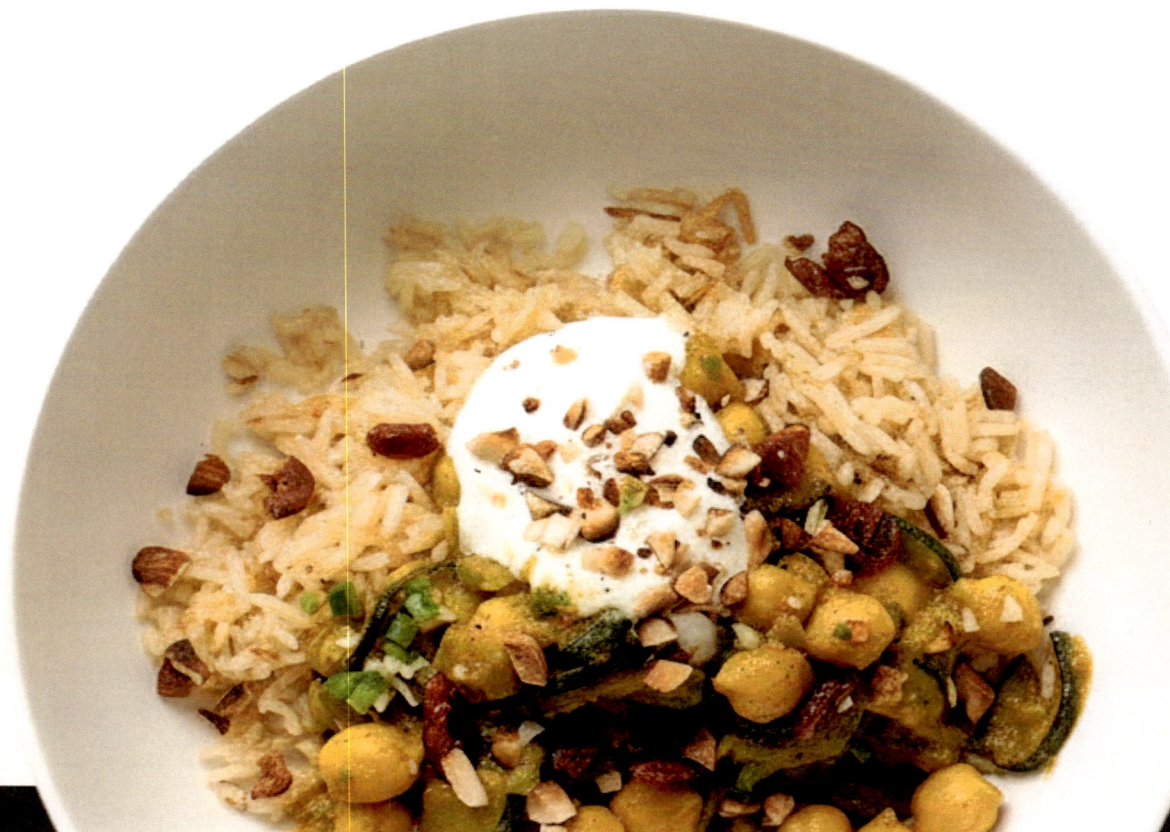

Sumac and harissa are key players in Middle Eastern and North African cuisines, offering tangy and spicy profiles that elevate even the simplest dishes. Harissa, originating from Tunisia, represents the region's love for bold, complex flavors. Sumac, derived from dried berries, has been a staple in Levantine cooking for centuries, known for its citrusy brightness. Maple syrup, a shout-out to Canadian and North American culinary traditions, reminds me of a sixth-grade science project where I tapped maple trees and learned how sap becomes syrup. This dish not only bridges continents but also tells a story of how traditional ingredients adapt and evolve in new contexts.

Quick Recipe Overview

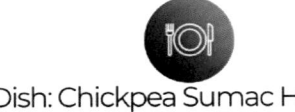

Dish: Chickpea Sumac Harissa Maple Salad

Prep Time: 15 minutes

Cook Time: 40 minutes

Serves: 4

Ingredients

FOR THE ROASTED VEGGIES:

1 sweet potato, diced: Adds natural sweetness and heartiness.
15 oz. can chickpeas: A staple in Middle Eastern cuisine, packed with protein.
2 large carrots, diced: Contributes crunch and a mild, earthy flavor.
1 red onion, peeled and diced: Enhances sweetness and depth when roasted.

FOR THE SALAD BASE:

Bundle of lettuce, kale, spinach, and/or mixed greens: A fresh foundation for the salad.
½ English cucumber, sliced into thin quarters: Adds a refreshing crunch.

FOR THE MARINADE:

2 tbsp. harissa paste: A fiery North African chili paste that brings heat and depth.
2 tbsp. sumac: A tangy spice commonly used in Middle Eastern dishes.
2 tbsp. maple syrup: Balances the spiciness with subtle sweetness.
Ground cinnamon, salt, and pepper to taste: Adds warmth and seasoning.

FOR THE DRESSING:

2 tbsp. tahini: A creamy sesame paste that enriches the dressing.
2 tbsp. sumac
2 tbsp. maple syrup
2 tbsp. harissa paste
2 tsp mustard: Adds a tangy, sharp flavor.
Aquafaba (reserved chickpea liquid) or water: A liquid to adjust the consistency.
Salt and pepper to taste

OPTIONAL TOPPINGS:

Goat cheese, walnuts, and/or raisins: Add creaminess, crunch, and sweetness.

FOR THE BREAD:

French baguette: A crispy accompaniment.
3 garlic cloves, minced
Olive oil: For pan-frying the bread.

Instructions

- **Preheat the Oven:**
    1. Preheat your oven to 425°F (220°C).
- **Prepare the Veggies:**
    1. Dice the sweet potato, carrots, and red onion. Place them in a mixing bowl.
- **Mix the Marinade:**
    In a small bowl, combine harissa paste, sumac, maple syrup, cinnamon, salt, and pepper.
    3. Pour the marinade over the diced veggies, tossing to coat evenly.
- **Roast the Veggies:**
    1. Spread the marinated veggies on a baking sheet in a single layer.
    2. Roast in the oven for 40 minutes, stirring them at the 20-minute mark to ensure even cooking.
- **Make the Dressing:**
    1. In a small jar, combine harissa paste, sumac, tahini, maple syrup, mustard, aquafaba (or water), salt, and pepper. Shake well to emulsify.
- **Assemble the Salad:**
    1. Toss the salad greens and cucumber with the dressing in a large bowl.
    2. Arrange in individual bowls, topping each with roasted veggies and optional goat cheese, walnuts, or raisins.
- **Prepare the Bread:**
    1. Spread minced garlic and olive oil on baguette slices.
    2. Pan-fry until golden and crispy. Serve alongside the salad. The crisp, garlicky bread provides a perfect contrast to the warm spices and creamy textures of the salad.

Pro Tips and Customizations

- Salad dressing bottle optional; however, many of us may already have one stored in the back of our pantries.

- For this flavorful spring salad, in a pinch, chili garlic paste may qualify as a partial substitute for Harissa paste.

This chickpea sumac harissa maple salad is a celebration of culinary diversity and creativity. With its vibrant flavors and nourishing ingredients, it is sure to become a favorite in your recipe rotation. Happy tossing!

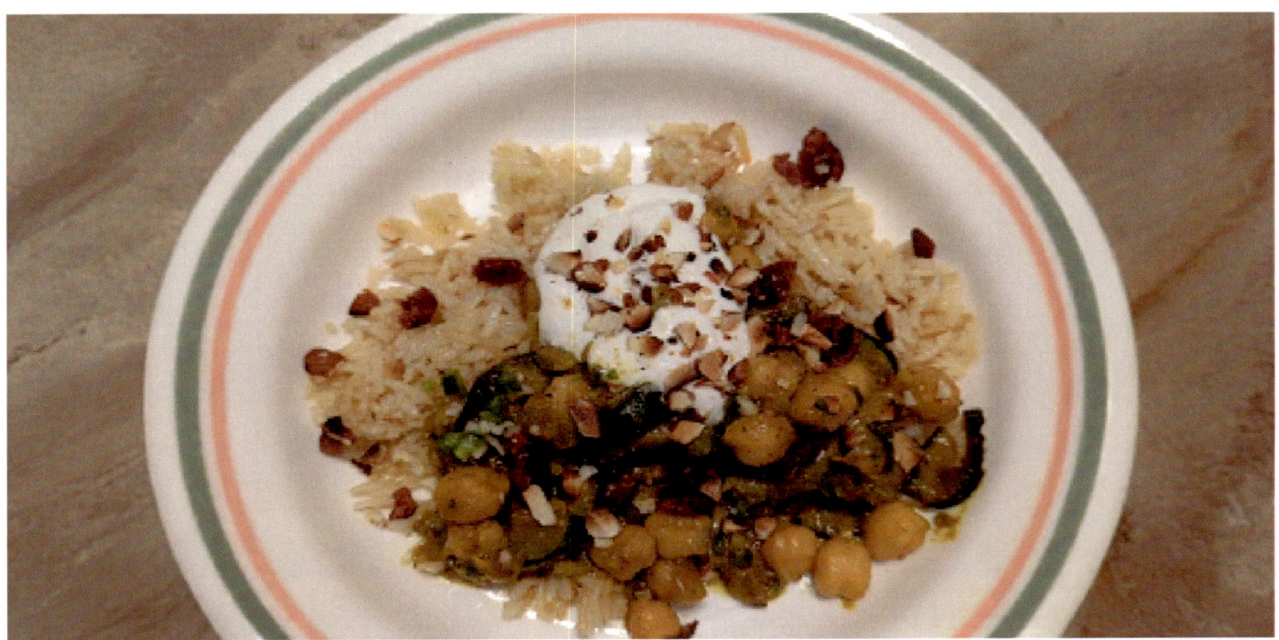

Corn and Avocado Salad:

A FRESH AND FLAVORFUL SUMMER DISH

Corn and avocado are ingredients that have significant historical and cultural backgrounds. Corn has been a staple in the Americas for thousands of years, originating as a crucial crop among Indigenous peoples. Avocado, another ancient crop from the same region, is known for its creamy texture and health benefits. Combining these two ingredients creates a dish that feels both timeless and current, reflecting the lasting influence of Mesoamerican cuisine on today's global palate.

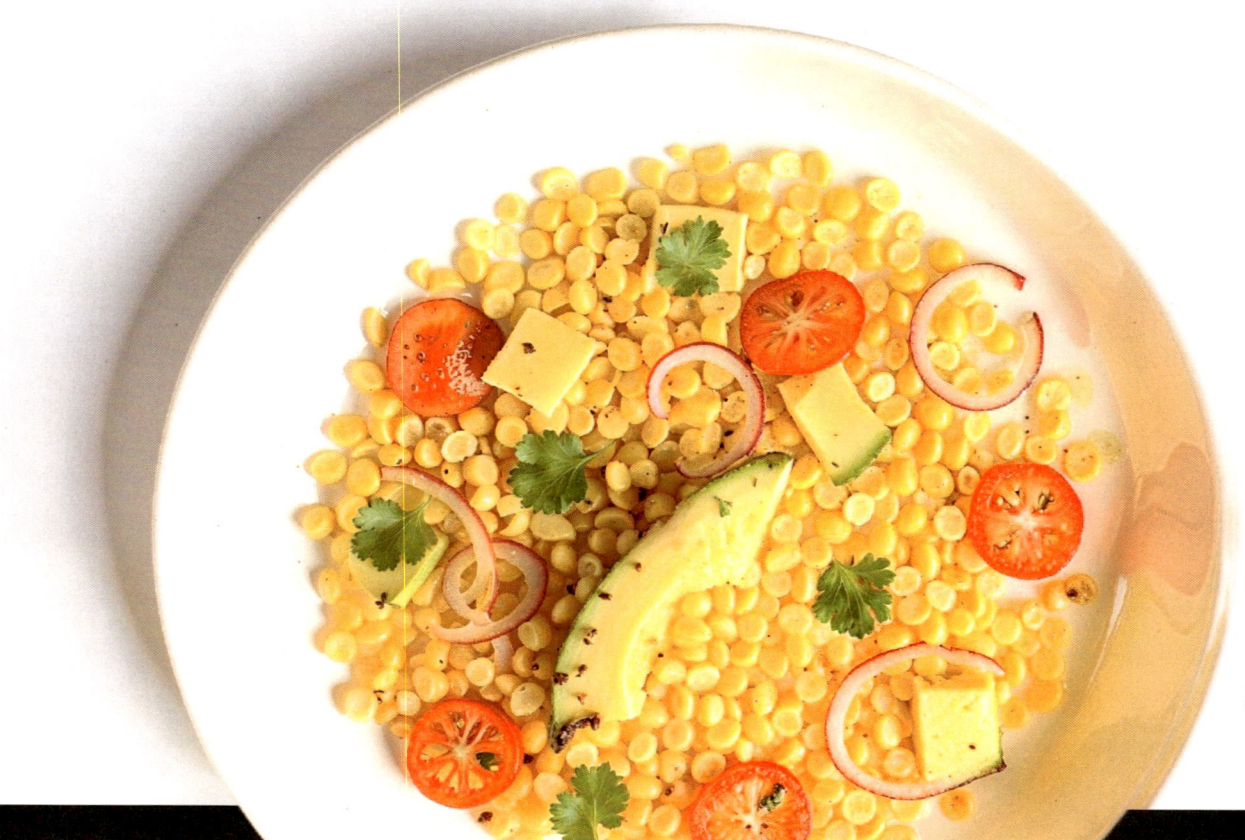

This corn and avocado salad is a light, refreshing dish perfect for warm days when you want something easy yet vibrant. Packed with juicy cherry tomatoes, creamy avocado, and tangy feta cheese, this salad makes a great side dish or even a main course. The addition of lime juice and arugula gives it a delightful zing and a hint of bitterness, balancing the sweetness of the corn. Avocados and corn have deep roots in Mesoamerican cuisine, where these ingredients have been staples for centuries. This dish celebrates those flavors with a modern twist, ideal for outdoor gatherings or quick weekday meals.

Ingredients

- 2 limes (zest and juice)
- 2 pints cherry tomatoes, halved
- 1 (32 oz.) bag frozen corn, thawed
- 2 large ripe avocados, cubed
- ½ cup extra virgin olive oil
- 2 tsp minced garlic
- 1 (5 oz.) bag baby arugula
- 1 (6 oz.) package crumbled feta cheese
- Salt and pepper, to taste

Instructions

- Zest and juice both limes.
- Halve the cherry tomatoes and place them in a large container with the thawed corn.

- Halve the avocados lengthwise, remove the pits, and cut them into cubes. Toss avocado cubes with 2 tablespoons of lime juice and add to the salad.

- In a separate container, mix the remaining lime juice, lime zest, olive oil, minced garlic, salt, and pepper. Shake well to combine.

- Store the salad, dressing, arugula, and crumbled feta in the fridge or a cooler until ready to serve. Keep ingredients separate until just before serving to maintain freshness and texture.

- Just before serving, toss the salad with the arugula and dressing, then garnish with crumbled feta cheese.

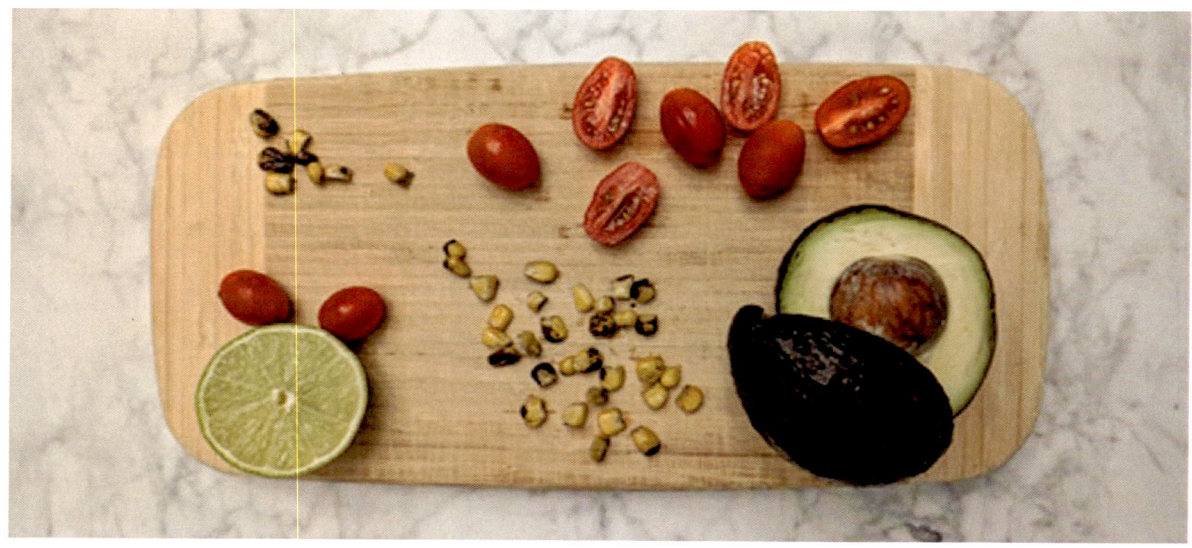

Pro Tips and Customizations

- For a spicier kick, add some diced jalapeño or a sprinkle of red pepper flakes.

- Substitute feta with goat cheese or queso fresco for a different flavor.

- If fresh corn is available, consider grilling it to add a smoky dimension to the salad.

I hope this corn and avocado salad brings a burst of freshness to your next meal!

Mains

Hearty Vegetable Chili:

A WARM AND WHOLESOME COMFORT DISH

Chili is a beloved dish with origins tracing back to the rich culinary history of Mexico and the southwestern United States. Traditionally made with meat, this vegetable version reflects the versatility and adaptability of chili to different diets and preferences. Beans, a key ingredient, have been a staple crop in many cultures for centuries due to their high protein content and heartiness. This vegetable chili showcases how plant-based ingredients can deliver the same satisfying experience as the classic dish, aligning with modern shifts towards plant-focused meals.

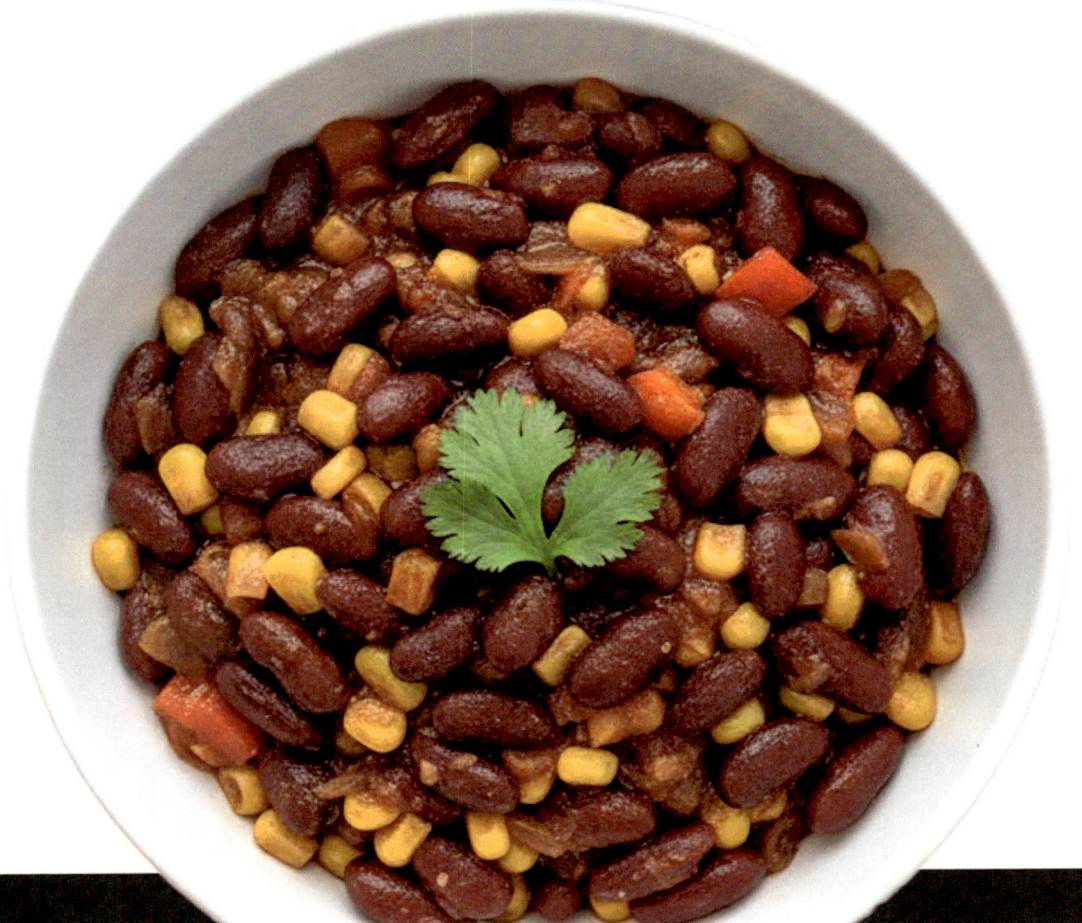

This hearty vegetable chili is a perfect one-pot meal that's packed with flavor and nutritious vegetables. With a blend of onions, peppers, zucchini, and mushrooms, this chili is a delicious, plant-based alternative to the classic meat chili. I love making this dish on cool evenings, as it fills the house with its warm feeling and aroma. It also offers a comforting meal that's both satisfying and versatile. Vegetable chili is also a great way to incorporate more veggies into your diet while still enjoying the rich, bold flavors of chili spices.

Ingredients

- 1 tablespoon oil
- 1 chopped onion
- ½ cup chopped bell pepper
- ½ chopped zucchini
- 1 cup corn
- ½ pound mushrooms, chopped
- 1 tablespoon chili powder
- ½ tablespoon ground cumin
- ½ tablespoon salt
- 1 ½ cups beans (such as black beans, kidney beans, or pinto beans)
- 16 oz. tomato sauce
- 1 cup water or vegetable broth
- Fresh cilantro, for garnish (optional)
- Cooked rice, for serving (optional)

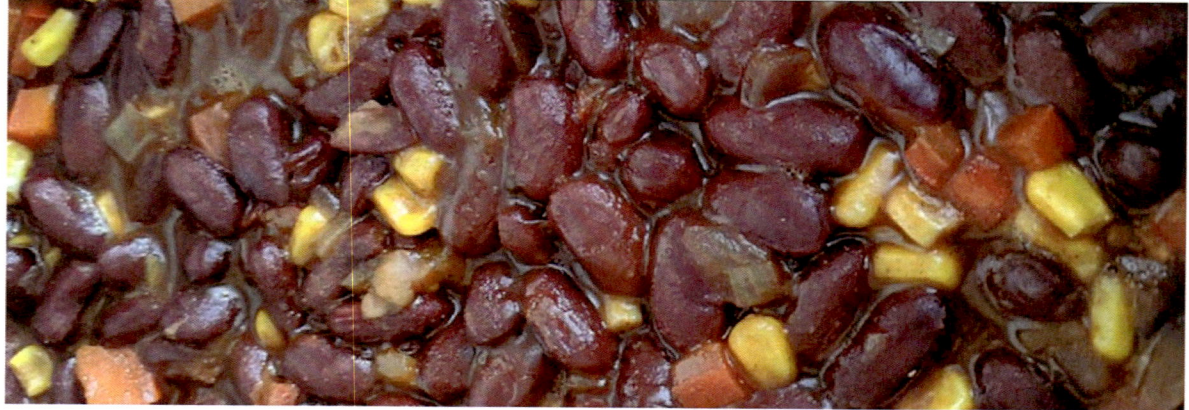

Instructions

1. Heat the oil in a large pot over medium heat. Add the chopped onions and bell peppers, and cook for about 3 minutes, until softened.

2. Add the zucchini, corn, and mushrooms, and cook for another 6 minutes, stirring occasionally.

3. Stir in the chili powder, cumin, and salt, and cook for 30 seconds to release the flavors.

4. Add the tomato sauce, beans, and water or vegetable broth. Stir well and bring the mixture to a boil.

5. Reduce the heat and let simmer, uncovered, for 20 minutes, stirring occasionally, until the chili thickens and flavors meld.

6. Serve hot, garnished with fresh cilantro and a side of cooked rice if desired.

Pro Tips and Customizations

- Add more vegetables like carrots or bell peppers for extra bulk and color.

- For a spicier kick, add a chopped jalapeño or a pinch of cayenne pepper.

- This chili is delicious served with toppings like shredded cheese, sour cream (my personal favorite), or avocado for extra richness.

> I hope you enjoy this hearty vegetable chili as much as I do! This vegetable chili is everything a good meal should be: hearty, comforting, full of flavor, and entirely plant-based.

Classic Tomato Soup with a Twist:

A MEDLEY OF FRESH INGREDIENTS AND VIBRANT FLAVORS

Tomato soup is a timeless comfort food, but this recipe elevates it with roasted red bell peppers, fresh basil, and a touch of chili heat. This dish has roots traced back to Mediterranean kitchens, where the abundance of fresh produce and bold seasonings inspires culinary magic. The simplicity of this soup allows the natural flavors of the ingredients to shine while showcasing techniques like blanching and grilling that enhance its depth. Whether served as a starter or a light meal, this tomato soup is both nourishing and flavorful, a perfect choice for savoring a bowl of culinary tradition.

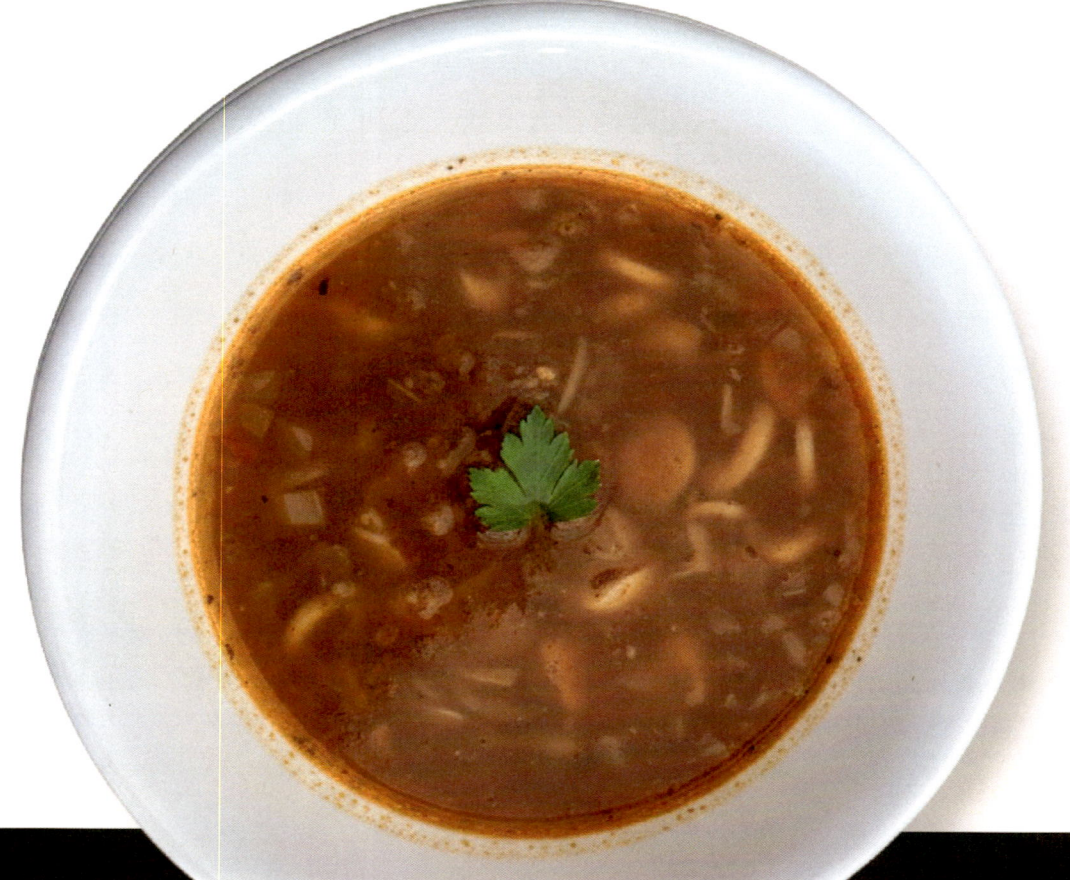

Tomato soup is a staple in cuisines around the world, with variations reflecting local ingredients and traditions. The use of ripe plum tomatoes and basil in this recipe highlights its Mediterranean influences, where fresh, simple flavors are celebrated. Grilled peppers add a smoky element often found in Spanish and Italian dishes, while the chili brings a collection of global spice traditions. This recipe embodies the adaptability of tomato soup, transforming humble ingredients into a vibrant and memorable dish. We eat tomato soup every Thanksgiving in my family, and this recipe is an adaptation of the one my aunt has served me for many years.

Quick Recipe Overview

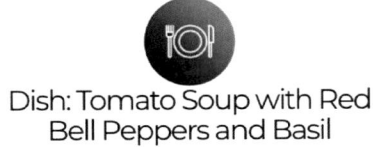

Dish: Tomato Soup with Red Bell Peppers and Basil

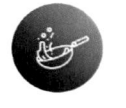

Prep Time: 15 minutes

Cook Time: 35 minutes

Serves: 4-6

Ingredients

FOR THE SOUP BASE:

- 15 ripe plum tomatoes: Sweet and juicy, ideal for a rich soup.
- 3 medium red bell peppers: Adds a smoky depth after grilling.
- ½ cup olive oil: Divided for cooking and finishing.
- 1 tbsp. chopped, seeded red chili: Brings a gentle heat.
- 2 cups vegetable broth: Provides a savory backbone.

FOR SEASONING:

- Salt and ground black pepper: To taste.
- 2 tbsp. red wine vinegar: Adds a tangy balance.

FOR GARNISH:

- 2 handfuls of fresh basil leaves: Aromatic and herbaceous.
- Additional red wine vinegar and olive oil: For finishing.

Instructions

- **Blanch the Tomatoes:**
  1. Score the tops of the tomatoes with a small "X."
  2. Blanch in boiling water for 20 seconds or until the skins start to loosen.
  3. Remove from the water, cool slightly, then peel and deseed. Chop the tomatoes finely and set aside.

- **Grill the Bell Peppers:**
  1. Grill the peppers whole over medium-high heat until charred on all sides.
  2. Transfer to a bowl and cover tightly to steam for 5 minutes. Peel off the skins, remove seeds, and finely chop the peppers.

- **Cook the Soup Base:**
  1. In a large saucepan, heat 2 tablespoons of olive oil over medium heat.
  2. Add the chopped red chili and a pinch of salt. Cook for 5 minutes.
  3. Stir in the garlic and cook for an additional 2 minutes.
  4. Add the chopped tomatoes and red bell peppers. Season with another pinch of salt and the red wine vinegar.
  5. Cook for 10 minutes, stirring occasionally.

- **Simmer the Soup:**
  1. Pour in the vegetable broth, stir well, and bring to a gentle simmer.
  2. Let the soup cook for 15 minutes, allowing the flavors to meld.
     (Bonus: I like to add fun-shaped pasta so the bowl of soup looks fun!)

- **Prepare the Basil Oil:**
  1. In a mortar and pestle, smash the basil leaves with a pinch of salt until a paste forms.
  2. Stir in the remaining olive oil and a dash of red wine vinegar. Set aside.

- **Finish and Serve:**
  1. Ladle the soup into bowls. Drizzle generously with the basil oil mixture.
  2. Serve warm with crusty bread or as a standalone dish.

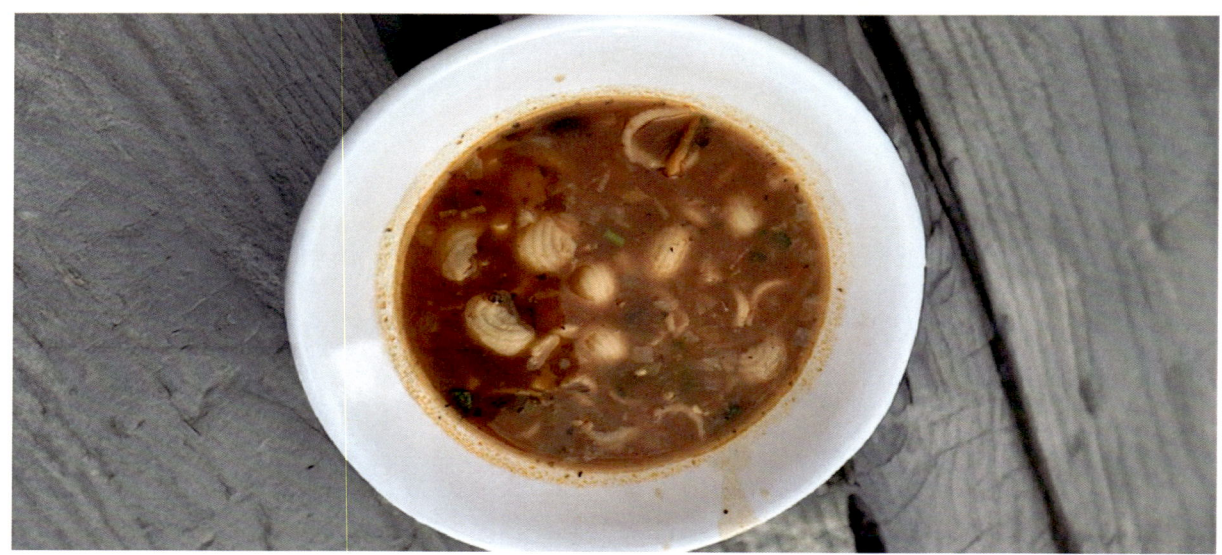

Pro Tips and Customizations

- For Extra Creaminess: Blend the soup and stir in a splash of heavy cream or coconut milk.

- Make it Vegan: This recipe is naturally vegan-friendly, but ensure your vegetable broth is free of animal products.

- Add Texture: Top with croutons, toasted pine nuts, or a dollop of ricotta cheese. Or, add pasta into the soup bowl to make it more appealing and fun to eat.

> This tomato soup recipe is a celebration of seasonal produce and time-honored techniques. Whether you're cooking for family or savoring a quiet meal, it offers a bowl of comfort steeped in history.

Classic Pizza with No Rise Dough and Fresh Tomato Sauce:

A QUICK AND EASY METHOD

Pizza has a rich cultural history in Italy, where it evolved from simple flatbreads into a beloved national dish. My best friend from second grade told me that early versions of pizza date back to ancient times, with flatbreads in Mediterranean cultures often topped with oils, herbs, and other ingredients. The modern pizza, however, originated in Naples in the 18th century. For the working class in Naples, pizza was a quick, inexpensive food sold by street vendors and small eateries, topped with ingredients that were affordable and flavorful, like tomatoes, which had recently been introduced to Europe from the Americas.

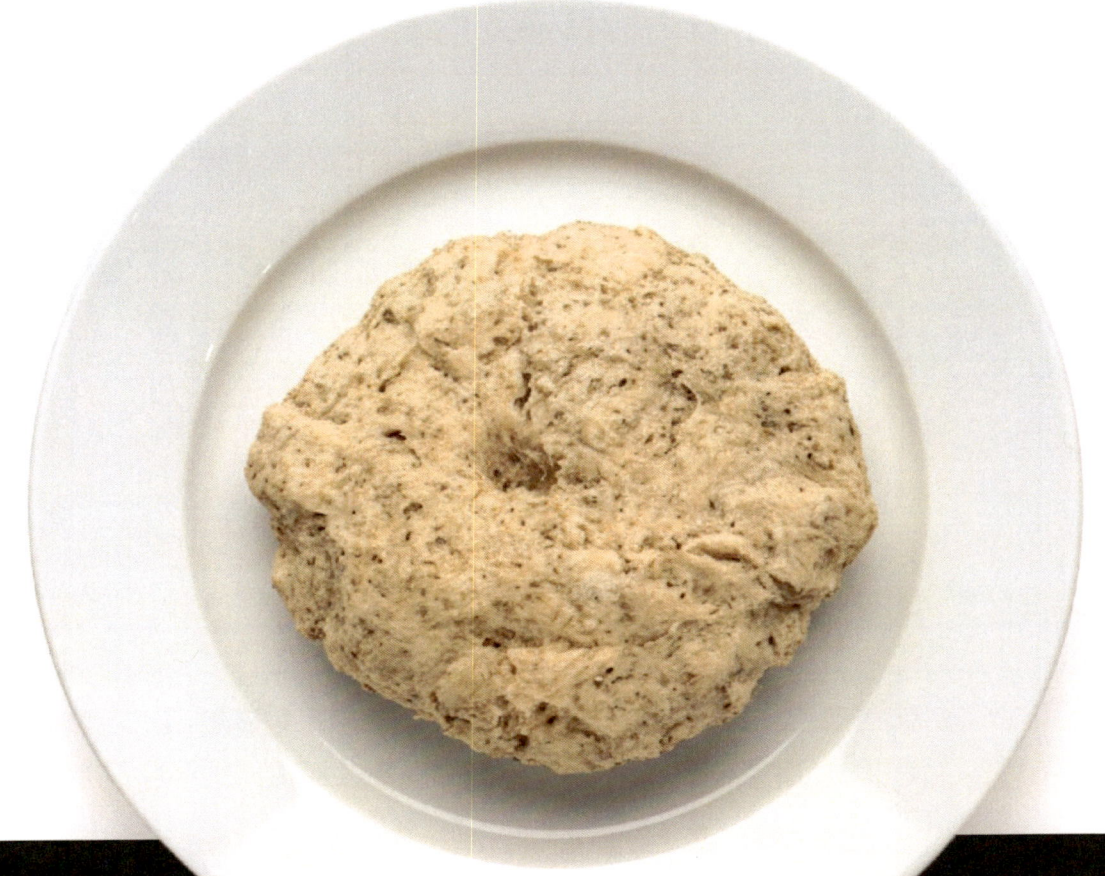

The creation of the Margherita pizza in 1889, made with tomatoes, mozzarella, and basil to represent the colors of the Italian flag, is often cited as a defining moment. Legend has it that Queen Margherita of Savoy favored this simple, patriotic pizza, helping it gain recognition beyond Naples. Today, pizza is celebrated worldwide, but Italians still take immense pride in their traditional methods, with specific guidelines in Naples for what constitutes a true Neapolitan pizza, emphasizing quality ingredients and artisanal preparation. Pizza in Italy is something that I enjoyed when visiting, and I hope to return again one day, perhaps even with my Italian friend from elementary school

Pizza is a dish that I love making with others. It is a hands-on activity, and can easily be served at a birthday celebration. Also, it can be customized during a small family gathering, where each chef can choose their own toppings. Pizza is often a fan favorite offering flavorful food that can be sliced up to serve both the minimally hungry and the famished appetite. Pizza dough is the key to making the perfect pizza, and this quick, no-rise recipe allows pizza to be made in a swift and easy manner while maintaining a crispy and satisfying crust base for toppings. In addition, a fresh sauce packs a punch with seasonal tomatoes, aromatic garlic, and fresh basil.

Plus, it is a fun, creative way to celebrate an assortment of seasonal veggies to put on top! Let kids get creative, experiment with toppings, and share their pizza masterpieces with family and friends!

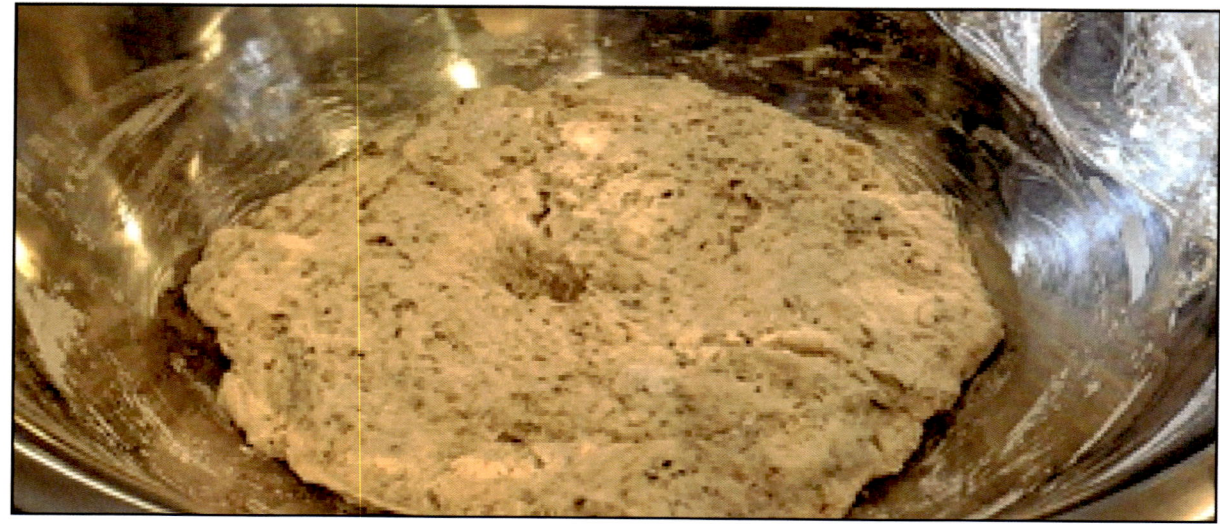

Ingredients

NO-RISE PIZZA DOUGH
1 cup warm water (110°F)
1 package active dry yeast (2 ¼ teaspoons)
1 teaspoon sugar
2 ½ cups all-purpose flour
2 tablespoons olive oil
1 teaspoon salt

FRESH TOMATO, GARLIC & BASIL SAUCE
3 tablespoons olive oil
3 cloves garlic, crushed
½ cup fresh parsley or basil leaves, chopped
6 medium to large fresh tomatoes, diced (or 2 pints cherry tomatoes, halved)
¼ teaspoon salt
½ cup cheese for topping (e.g., grated pecorino, goat cheese, burrata, or fresh mozzarella)

Instructions

To Make the Dough:

1. Preheat the oven to 450°F.
2. In a medium bowl, mix warm water, yeast, and sugar. Let it sit for about 10 minutes, until the mixture becomes bubbly.
3. Add flour, olive oil, and salt. Knead by hand or use a mixer with a dough hook until smooth.
4. Turn the dough onto a lightly floured surface, press with the palm of your hand, and shape into a pizza base. Place on a pizza pan and set aside while you prepare the sauce and toppings.

To Make the Fresh Tomato Sauce:

1. Lightly crush garlic cloves, sprinkle with salt, and chop.
2. In a medium saucepan, warm olive oil over medium heat. Add garlic and cook until golden.
3. Add tomatoes, cooking until they release juices and break down, about 10 minutes. If the sauce is dry, add ¼ cup of water and cook for 5 more minutes.
4. Remove from heat, sprinkle with fresh basil or parsley, and let cool slightly.

Assemble the Pizza:

1. Spread the fresh tomato sauce onto the pizza dough.
2. Add cheese and any additional toppings of your choice.
3. Bake in the oven for 12-15 minutes, until the crust is golden and the cheese is melted.

Pro Tips and Customizations

- For a grill option, cook the pizza dough on a preheated grill, then add toppings and cook until the cheese melts.

- Try different cheeses like burrata or goat cheese for unique flavor combinations.

- Add veggies like bell peppers, onions, or arugula to make it your own.

> To me, pizza embodies the value of simplicity and quality. I actually like mine without cheese and typically seek out using fresh, local ingredients. Next time you make pizza, consider how you are eating a dish that began centuries ago and how it brings you joy and flavor, no matter your age.

Saffron Linguine:

THE GOLDEN SPICE MEETS A PANTRY CLASSIC

Saffron linguine is proof that a simple dish can transport you to another world with just a few key ingredients. This recipe takes a humble pantry staple, linguine, and elevates it with the magic of saffron, often referred to as the "golden spice."

For centuries, saffron has been one of the most prized spices in the world, celebrated for its vibrant hue, unique aroma, and storied history. Originating in the Middle East, saffron has traveled across continents, gracing dishes from Persian rice to Spanish paella. In this recipe, saffron combines with cream, parmesan, and the natural sweetness of corn (a gift from the Americas) to create a dish that feels both luxurious and comforting.

Saffron's history is as rich as its color. First cultivated in ancient Persia, it was traded along the Silk Road, becoming a symbol of luxury and health. In medieval Europe, saffron was so valuable that it was used as currency and even sparked wars.

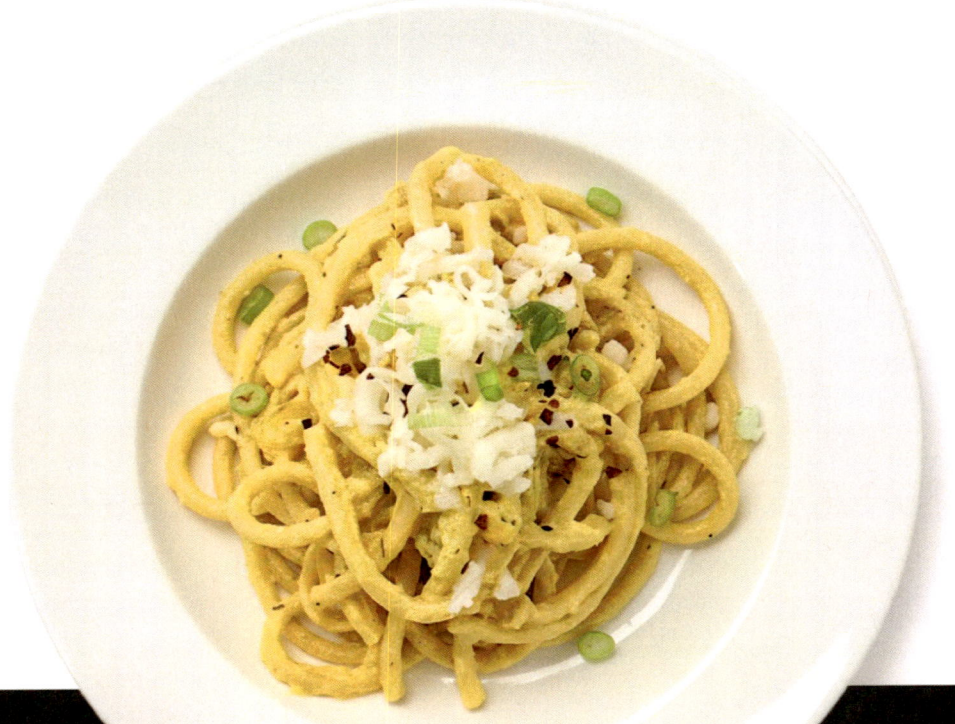

The use of saffron in pasta dishes like this linguine is a reflection of global culinary fusion. Italian cuisine embraced saffron through its connections to the Mediterranean spice trade, where it became a key ingredient in dishes like Milanese risotto. Today, saffron remains one of the most expensive spices by weight, not only for its labor-intensive production but also for its enduring cultural significance.

Whether you're hosting a dinner party or simply treating yourself, this saffron linguine brings a touch of history and indulgence to your table.

> This creamy saffron linguine balances the richness of butter and cream with the bright flavors of basil and lemon. Ready in 20 minutes, it's an elegant way to make the most of pantry ingredients.

Ingredients

1 box of linguine pasta – A staple of Italian cuisine dating back to the 12th century.

1 ½ tbsp. unsalted butter, divided – Adds richness and a velvety texture.

1 ½ tbsp. extra virgin olive oil – A cornerstone of Mediterranean cooking.

2 tbsp. minced shallot – A subtle allium with origins in central Asia.

3 garlic cloves, thinly sliced – Used globally for its flavor and health benefits.

1 small pinch saffron threads (8–10 threads) – The "golden spice," valued for its rarity and history.

¾ cup milk – Adds creaminess without heaviness.

2 oz. freshly grated Parmesan cheese – A hallmark of Italian cuisine, aged for depth of flavor.

Salt and cracked black pepper, to taste

Fresh basil leaves, garnish – A fragrant herb used since ancient times for both flavor and healing.

Instructions

1. Cook the linguine: Fill a large pot with water, add a handful of salt, and bring to a boil. Add the linguine, stirring occasionally, and cook until al dente (6–8 minutes). Reserve 1 cup of pasta water before draining the linguine.

2. Prepare the saffron-infused sauce: Heat 1 ½ tbsp. butter and olive oil in a large skillet over medium-high heat. Add shallots and garlic, sautéing for 2–3 minutes until fragrant. Season with salt.

3. Simmer the saffron: Add the reserved pasta water and saffron threads to the skillet. Let the mixture simmer and reduce by half. The saffron will release its golden hue and earthy aroma. Note: Saffron threads are derived from the stigmas of the crocus sativus flower. Harvesting requires immense labor: over 70,000 flowers to produce just one pound of saffron.

4. Create the creamy base: Stir in the milk and parmesan cheese, letting the sauce thicken slightly. Season with salt and pepper to taste.

5. Combine the pasta and sauce: Add the linguine to the skillet and toss to coat in the saffron cream. Adjust seasoning as needed.

6. Serve and garnish: Plate the pasta and top with freshly grated parmesan and basil leaves for a fragrant finish. Serve immediately.

Pro Tips and Customizations

- Swap out linguine for spaghetti or fettuccine if that's what you have on hand.

- For a citrusy twist, add a splash of fresh lemon juice to the sauce.

- No saffron? Turmeric can mimic its color, but the flavor will differ.

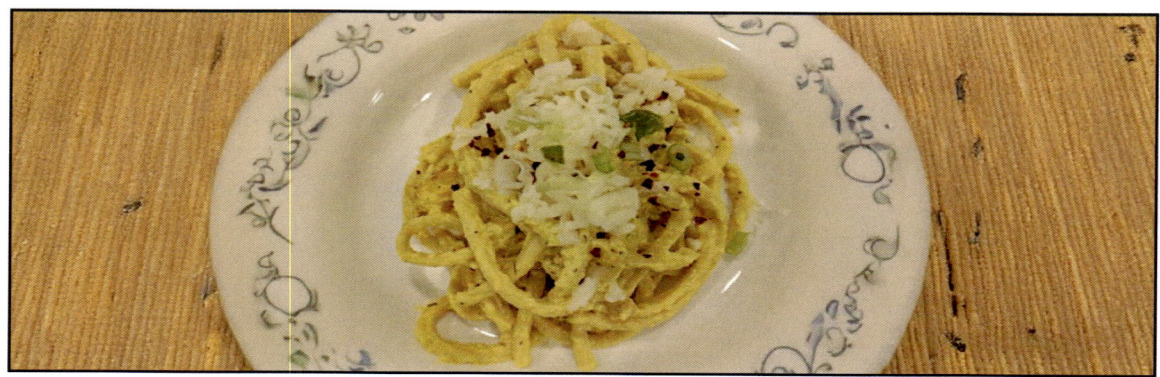

I hope you enjoy using saffron in your recipes. Typically, I see saffron used as an ingredient in dessert dishes, but this recipe brings saffron into the main meal! I hope you can customize the use of saffron in your food, so long as you don't get sticker shock at just how pricey getting this spice is!

Spaghetti Squash with Italian Style Tomato Sauce

Many of us seek the comforting embrace of hearty, nourishing meals. Spaghetti squash, with its magical ability to transform into delicate strands resembling pasta, has captured the hearts of food enthusiasts worldwide. But did you know that this humble squash has a rich cultural and historical background? Native to the Americas, squash varieties were staples for Indigenous peoples long before European settlers arrived. This recipe, pairing spaghetti squash with Italian-inspired tomato sauce, is a meeting point of culinary traditions that span continents. I hope you will see how these ingredients reflect cultural exchanges while creating a dish that's both nutritious and satisfying.

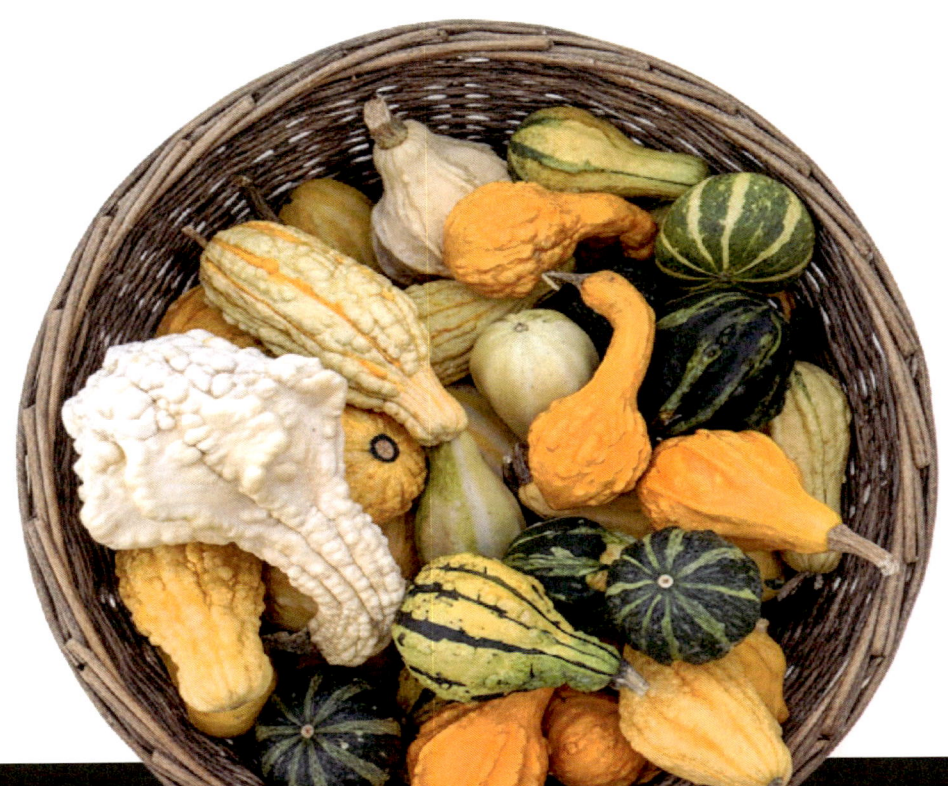

Spaghetti squash's history is rooted in the agricultural practices of Indigenous peoples in the Americas, where squash was cultivated alongside corn and beans. Its later adoption into global cuisines highlights the interconnectedness of food traditions. Tomatoes, native to Central and South America, were initially met with suspicion in Europe but are now synonymous with Italian cooking. This recipe symbolizes the fusion of these culinary journeys, showcasing how food transcends borders to bring diverse flavors together.

Quick Recipe Overview

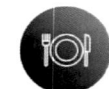

Dish: Spaghetti Squash with Italian-Style Tomato Sauce

Prep Time: 10 minutes

Cook Time: 55 minutes

Serves: 2 as a side or 1 as a main

Ingredients

- **For the Squash:**

1. ½ medium spaghetti squash: A winter squash originating from the Americas, it has become a favorite in many cuisines for its versatility.
2. 1 tbsp. extra virgin olive oil: Central to Mediterranean cooking, olive oil adds richness and ties the dish to its Italian inspiration.

- **For the Sauce:**

1. 1 cup diced onion: Adds sweetness and depth; onions are a staple in global cuisines.
2. ⅛ Tsp sea salt: Harvested from the sea, it's an ancient seasoning used in preservation and flavoring.
3. ¼ tsp ground black pepper: Indigenous to India, black pepper became a prized spice in Europe.
4. 1 clove garlic, minced: Revered in culinary traditions worldwide for its bold flavor.
5. 8 oz. Italian-style diced tomatoes (with juices): A cornerstone of Italian cooking, tomatoes originated in the Americas and were embraced in Europe after the Columbian Exchange.
6. ¼ cup vegetable broth: Enhances the sauce's flavor and keeps it light.
7. 1 tbsp. extra virgin olive oil (for serving): Drizzled for extra richness.

Instructions

- **Prepare the Squash:**

Preheat the oven to 350°F (175°C).

Cut the spaghetti squash lengthwise in half, avoiding the stem.

Place one half, cut side up, in a baking dish. Bake for about 45 minutes or until the flesh is easily pierced with a knife.

- **Cook the Onions:**
  1. Heat 1 tbsp. olive oil in a medium skillet over medium heat.
  2. Add diced onions, half the salt, and half the pepper. Stir to coat and cook for 10 minutes until softened.
- **Make the Sauce:**
  1. Add the diced tomatoes, vegetable broth, and minced garlic to the skillet with onions. Stir well.
  2. Cover and let the mixture simmer for 10 minutes, allowing the flavors to meld.
- **Shred the Squash:**
  1. Remove the baked squash from the oven and let it cool slightly.
  2. Scoop out the seeds and discard them.
  3. Use a fork to shred the squash flesh, dragging it lengthwise to create spaghetti-like strands.
- **Assemble and Serve:**
  1. Place the shredded squash on a serving dish.
  2. Spoon the tomato sauce over the squash, mixing gently to combine.
  3. Drizzle with the remaining 1 tbsp. olive oil. Adjust seasoning with the remaining salt and pepper if needed.

Pro Tips and Customizations

- Customize the Sauce: Add fresh basil, oregano, or red chili flakes for extra layers of flavor.

- Make it Cheesy: Sprinkle grated Parmesan or nutritional yeast for a creamy finish.

Food tells stories, and this spaghetti squash with Italian-style tomato sauce is a testament to the global nature of culinary traditions. Whether you're drawn to its historical roots or its nutritional benefits, this dish offers a delightful experience. Take a moment to savor the transformation of this tasty vegetable and keep the conversation around the dinner table about food and culture alive!

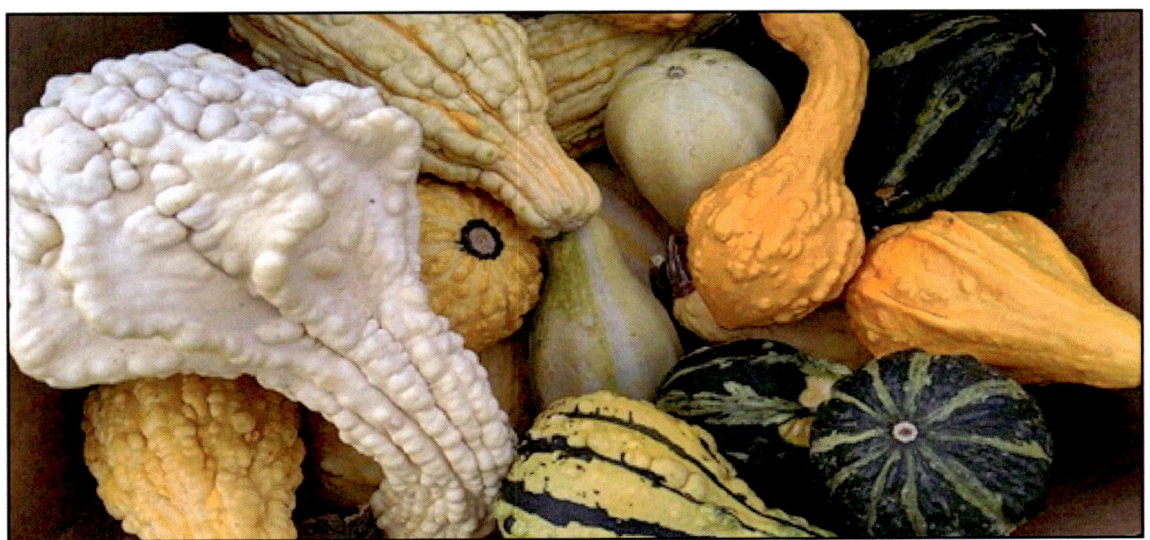

Lemon Garlic Orzo with Veggies:

A MEDITERRANEAN MEDLEY OF FLAVOR AND HISTORY

Orzo, while technically a pasta, is shaped to resemble rice and is often mistaken for a grain. It hails from the Mediterranean, particularly Italian and Greek cuisines, where it's been used in soups, salads, and side dishes for generations. The word orzo means "barley" in Italian, reflecting the grain-like texture it brings to dishes.

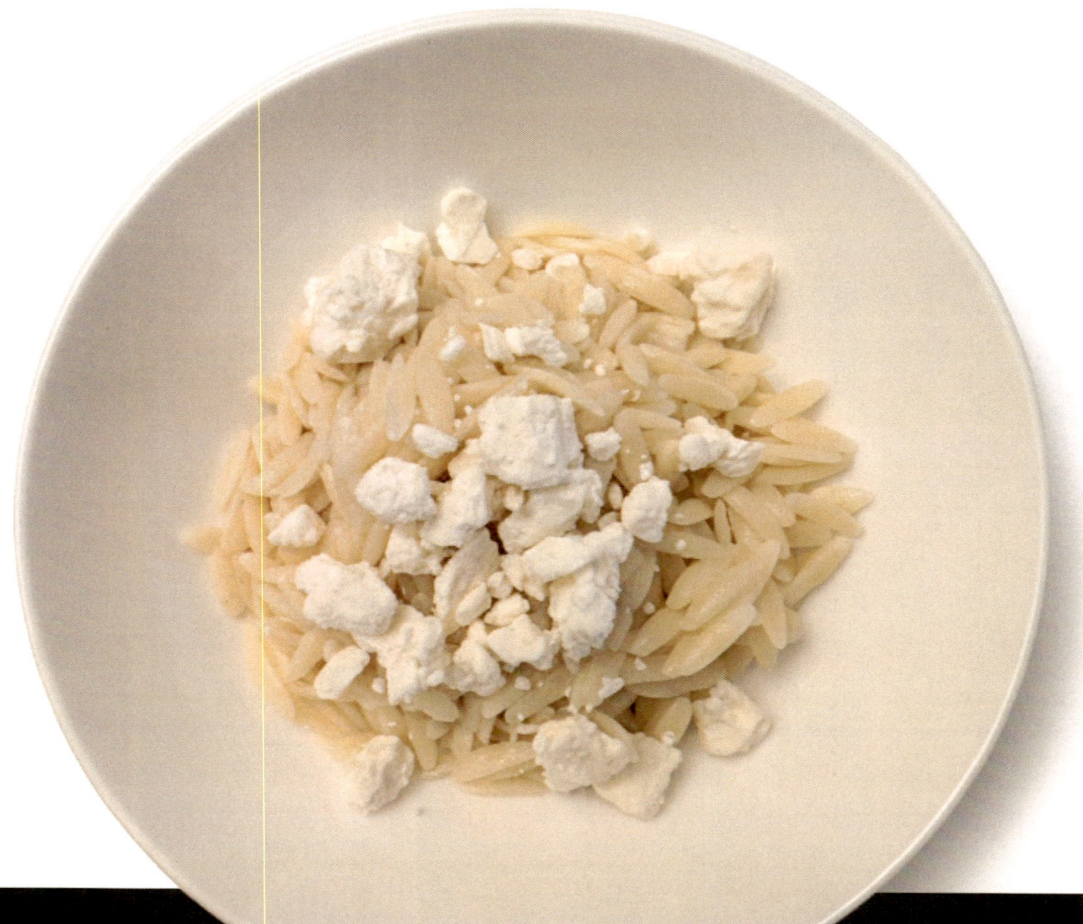

Garlic, used both fresh and powdered here, has been revered for its culinary and medicinal properties for over 5,000 years. Ancient Egyptians used it to nourish pyramid builders, while Greeks and Romans believed it gave soldiers strength. Its use across the Mediterranean is tied to both practicality and ritual, an aromatic cornerstone of the regional diet.

Feta cheese and olive oil, two more Mediterranean staples, offer a lens into the heart-healthy traditions of one of the world's oldest culinary regions. Together, they create the signature balance of briny, creamy, and earthy that defines the cuisine.

Finally, lemon, symbolic of cleansing and preservation in both food and culture, brightens the dish while reflecting the ancient agricultural legacy of the Mediterranean citrus belt.

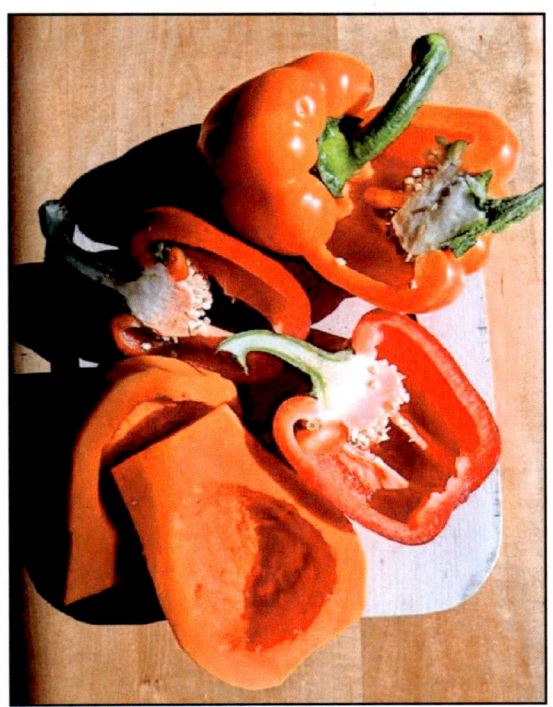

This lemon garlic orzo with veggies is a sun-kissed bowl of bright, bold flavor with a simple and satisfying way to celebrate the Mediterranean pantry. Roasted seasonal vegetables meet golden orzo pasta, bound together by garlic, lemon, and feta for a dish that feels as restorative as it is flavorful. Each bite offers a satisfying mix of citrusy brightness, garlicky depth, and creamy feta tang.

Though it reads like a modern wellness recipe, this dish is steeped in tradition. This dish not only satisfies the palate but also supports heart health with antioxidant-rich veggies and olive oil. From the ancient Greek use of orzo-like grains to the Roman reverence for garlic, each component carries centuries of culinary heritage.

Ingredients

1 cup red or yellow bell pepper, cubed

1 lb. asparagus, trimmed and cut into 2-inch pieces

12 oz. cherry tomatoes

2 tsp minced garlic (or garlic powder to taste)

3 tbsp. olive oil

½ tsp salt

½ tsp black pepper

1 cup orzo pasta

1½ cups vegetable broth

Feta cheese, crumbled (to taste)

Fresh lemon juice (to taste)

Optional: fresh diced tomatoes for garnish

Instructions

Roast the Vegetables

1. Preheat the oven to 425°F. Line two sheet pans with parchment paper.
2. Spread bell pepper, asparagus, and cherry tomatoes on the pans.
3. Drizzle with 2 Tbsp. olive oil, sprinkle with salt and pepper, and toss to coat.
4. Roast for 35–40 minutes until veggies are tender and lightly caramelized.

Prepare the Orzo

1. In a saucepan, heat 1 Tbsp. oil and lightly toast the orzo until golden.
2. Add vegetable broth, cover, and simmer on low heat for 15 minutes, or until liquid is absorbed and orzo is tender.

- **Combine and Season**
1. In a sauté pan, mix the cooked orzo and roasted vegetables.
2. Add minced garlic (or garlic powder), salt, pepper, and lemon juice to taste. Stir well.
3. Top with crumbled feta cheese and, optionally, fresh chopped tomatoes before serving.

Pro Tips and Customizations

- For a gluten-free option, substitute orzo with rice-shaped gluten-free pasta or cooked millet.
- Add chickpeas or lentils for extra protein.
- Stir in fresh herbs like dill or parsley for brightness.
- Serve warm or cold.

This recipe is not just a meal, it is a snapshot of Mediterranean food philosophy: fresh ingredients, seasonal produce, simple prep, and nourishing balance. I used to eat this dish with all the vegetables on the side, so my bowl was just a mixture of white and beige, but at least this way I could enjoy the flavor of the cheese. Nevertheless, eating the rainbow is a common phrase in my home. Try your own version and then pause to savor what your orzo story looks and tastes like!

Paneer Burgers:

CRISPY, SPICED, AND VEGETARIAN-FRIENDLY

These crispy paneer burgers are more than just a vegetarian meal because they are a cross-cultural celebration of tradition and innovation. Built around paneer, the fresh Indian cheese with ancient roots.

This recipe takes inspiration from street food and home cooking across South Asia and reimagines it in the familiar form of the American burger. With a spiced potato-paneer patty and bold herbs, this dish blends history, texture, and flavor into every bite. Expect a crisp exterior with warm spices, a soft interior, and fresh herbal notes from the cilantro. A special shout-out to my loving masis (aunts) from New Jersey who taught my family how to make this delicious recipe.

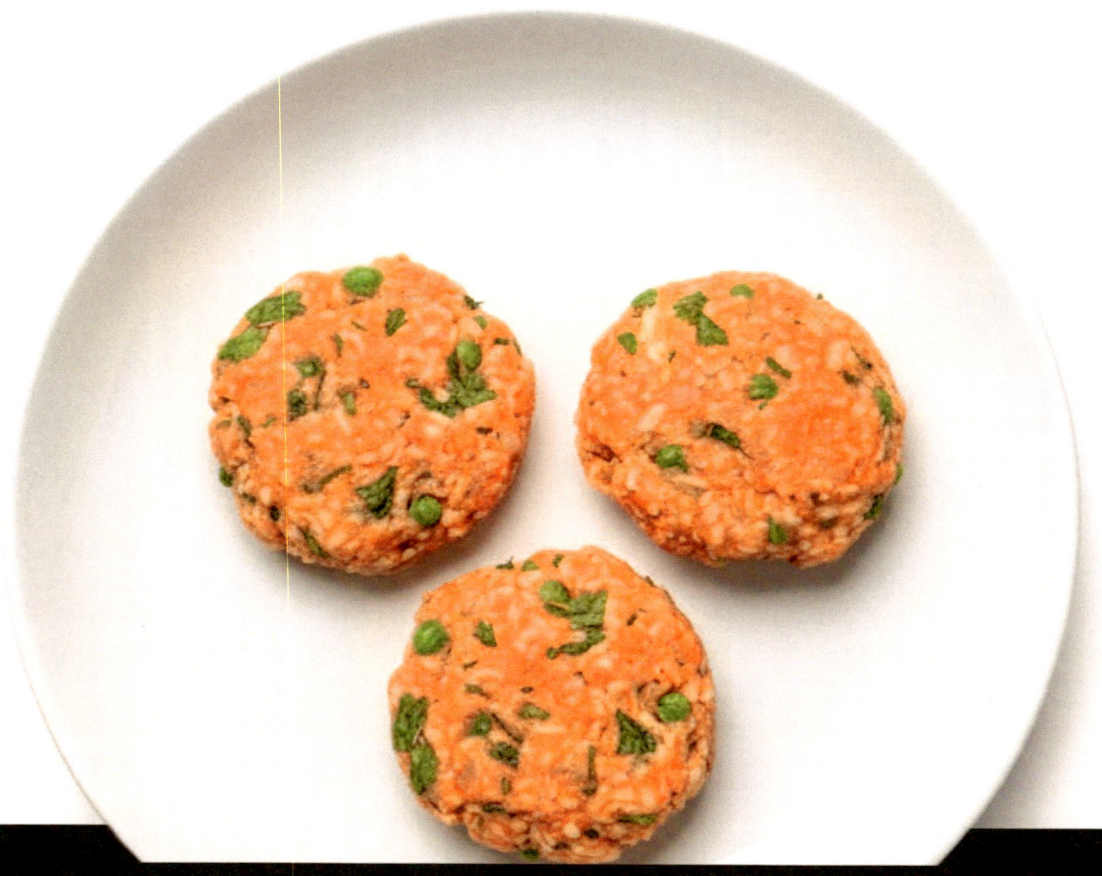

Paneer, a fresh, non-melting cheese, has been part of the Indian subcontinent's food culture for over 2,000 years. Its name likely derives from the Persian panir, introduced during centuries of trade and conquest in South Asia. Paneer is made by curdling milk with lemon juice or vinegar, which is a method used for centuries in home kitchens and temple kitchens alike. Unlike aged cheeses from Europe, paneer's simplicity and versatility made it a cornerstone of vegetarian diets.

The spices in this burger, including cumin, coriander, and red pepper flakes, reflect India's role as a historical hub of the spice trade, where flavor has long carried symbolic, medicinal, and economic weight.

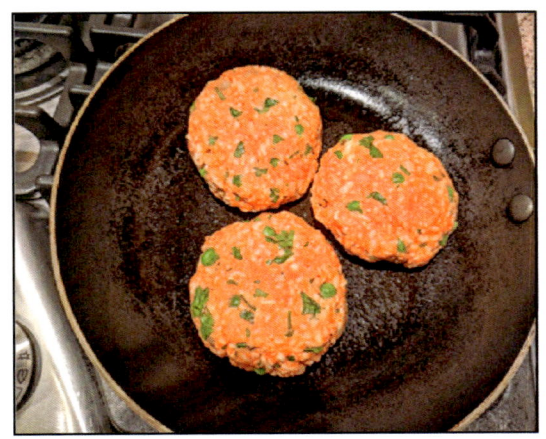

Whether served at a casual gathering or as a weeknight comfort dish, these burgers remind us that culinary fusion is often born from migration, adaptation, and creativity.

Ingredients

FOR THE PATTIES:
1 lb. yellow potatoes, peeled and cubed
6 oz. low-fat paneer, grated
1 tsp red pepper flakes

1 tsp garlic powder
1 tsp onion powder
1 tsp ground cumin
1 tsp ground coriander
1 tsp salt (or to taste)
1 cup loosely packed cilantro leaves, finely chopped
3 Tbsp. vegetable cooking oil
Bread crumbs (for coating)

Instructions

- **Boil the Potatoes**
  1. In a large pot, boil peeled and cubed yellow potatoes in salted water until fork-tender. Drain and transfer to a large mixing bowl.

- **Mash and Mix**
  1. Mash the potatoes until smooth with no large chunks remaining.
  2. Add grated paneer, red pepper flakes, garlic powder, onion powder, cumin, coriander, salt, and chopped cilantro. Mix thoroughly.

- **Form Patties**
  1. Use a ½ cup measuring cup to scoop out the mixture. Form into even-sized patties.
  2. Coat each patty with bread crumbs for extra crispiness.

Instructions

Pan Fry

1. Heat oil in a large skillet over medium heat. Once hot, pan-fry patties in batches for about 6 minutes per side, or until golden brown and crispy. Add more oil as needed between batches.

Assemble and Serve

1. Serve patties on toasted hamburger buns with your choice of condiments. Suggested
2. toppings: green chutney or mustard, sliced red onion, cucumber, tomato, fresh greens, and jalapeños for extra spice.

By placing the patty between burger buns and topping it with chutneys and veggies, this dish bridges two worlds: the grab-and-go burger culture of the West and the spice-laden vegetarian traditions of the East.

Pro Tips and Customizations

- Use sweet potatoes for a twist on the patty base.
- Swap in Greek yogurt-based sauce instead of mustard for a tangy flavor.
- Bake the patties instead of frying for a lighter option.
- Add peas, carrots, or shredded beets to the patty for extra color and nutrition.
- Try it with tamarind chutney or a yogurt-cilantro sauce.
- Use whole-wheat buns or lettuce wraps for a low-carb option.

I hope these crispy paneer patties bring something new to your table! They're simple to make, full of flavor, and easy to prepare ahead of meal time. Feel free to play with the spices and toppings of your own choice!

Potato Shaak:

Shaak is deeply rooted in Gujarati-Indian culture, where vegetarianism is not just a dietary preference but often a religious and philosophical commitment. Influences from Hinduism and the arid climate of western India have led to a cuisine that emphasizes spices, legumes, seasonal vegetables, and balanced flavors.

Potatoes, now a staple in Indian households, were introduced by Portuguese traders in the 17th century. Since then, they've been adopted into countless regional dishes like this one.

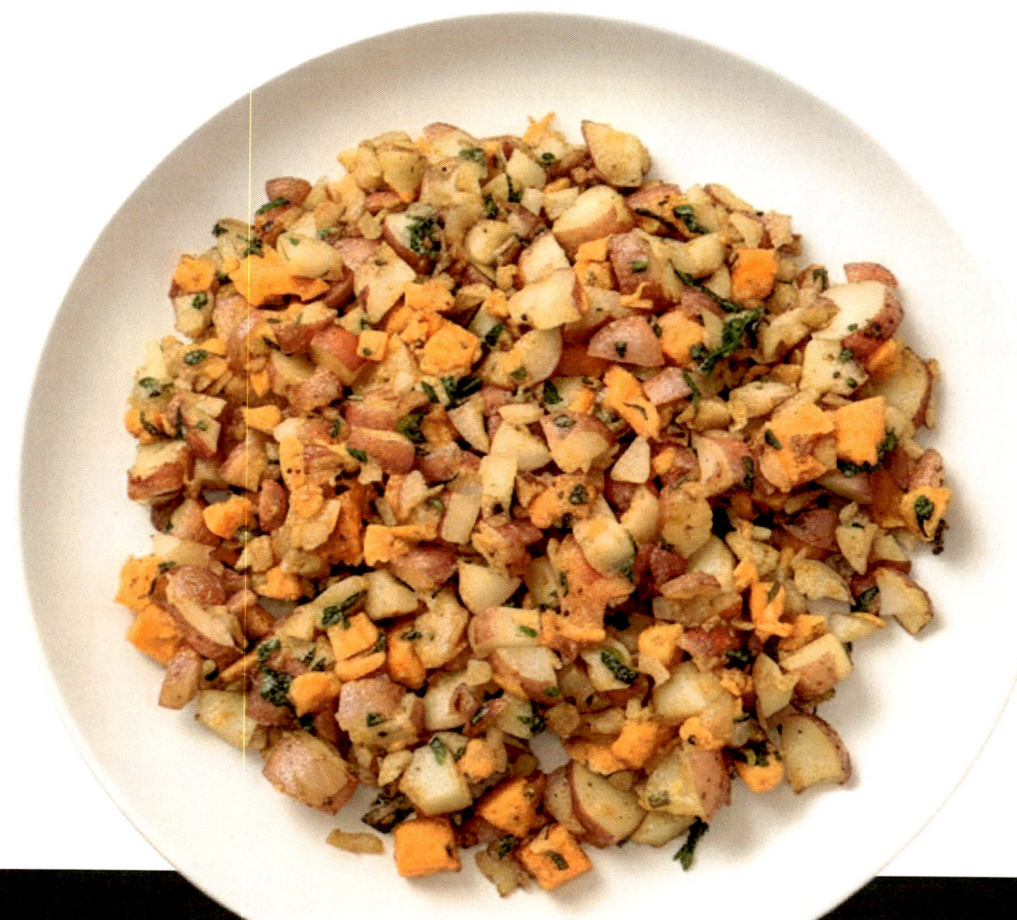

Cumin seeds, used here to temper the oil, have been cultivated in India since antiquity. Their warm, earthy flavor is a cornerstone of Indian "tadkas", or tempering methods that date back thousands of years.

The option to substitute tomatoes with cashews and raisins reflects both the seasonal adaptability of Gujarati cooking and the tradition of sweet-savory contrasts, which is a hallmark of my own family's variation. This version adds richness and a touch of sweetness.

Even the balance of lemon juice and sugar illustrates the Gujarati palate's famous love of a vibrant mix of tangy, spicy, and sweet that excites all parts of the tongue.

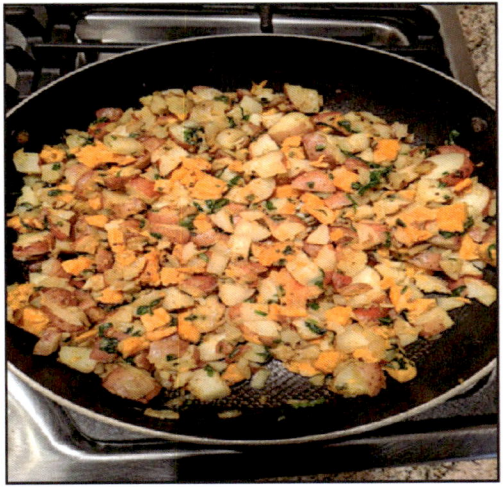

Potato Shaak is a humble yet deeply flavorful Gujarati-style curry made with mashed or cubed potatoes simmered in a fragrant mix of spices, onions, and either tomatoes or dried fruit. It is quick to make and big on comfort, a perfect example of how simplicity and tradition come together on the everyday Indian plate, with a mixture of warmth, heat, tang and sweet.

Ingredients

4 medium potatoes – boiled, peeled, and cubed or mashed

1 tsp crushed garlic

A small pinch of fresh ginger (grated or crushed)

2–3 green chilies, finely chopped

1 tomato, finely chopped (or substitute with cashews and raisins for a richer, festive version)

1 onion, finely chopped

½ tsp turmeric powder

1 tsp cumin seeds

½ tsp sugar

1 tsp lemon juice

Salt to taste

Fresh coriander leaves, chopped (for garnish)

1 tsp oil for cooking

Instructions

- **Prep the Potatoes**
  1. Boil potatoes until very soft. Peel and either cube them or mash roughly, depending on the desired texture.

- **Make the Base Masala**
  1. In a pan, heat oil over a medium flame. Add cumin seeds and let them splutter.
  2. Add chopped green chilies and onions. Sauté until onions turn golden.
  3. Add chopped tomato (or dried fruit if substituting), and cook down until soft and slightly saucy.

- **Spice it Up**
  1. Stir in ginger, garlic, turmeric, and salt. Cook for 2–3 minutes until aromatic.

- **Add the Potatoes**
  1. Add the mashed or cubed potatoes to the pan. Mix thoroughly so they absorb all the flavors.
  2. Cook for a few more minutes to let the shaak thicken slightly.

- **Finish with Sweet & Sour**
  1. Stir in the sugar and lemon juice. Adjust seasoning if needed.
  2. Garnish with fresh coriander before serving.

Pro Tips and Customizations

- Prefer a richer version? Use ghee instead of oil.

- Add tomatoes, peas, or sweet potato for a little variation.

- No chilies? Add a pinch of red chili powder or skip for a milder flavor.

- Serve with roti, puri, or rice for a classic Gujarati meal.

Potato shaak is the kind of dish that adapts to what you have, how you feel, and who you are feeding. Passed down through generations, it is both practical and poetic, full of flavor, heritage, and care. Make it your own, knowing that shaak has many variations and voices.

Khichdi:

THE ANCIENT INDIAN COMFORT FOOD THAT NOURISHES BODY AND SOUL

Khichdi is arguably one of the oldest continuously prepared dishes in South Asia, with references in Ayurvedic texts dating back over 2,000 years. A simple preparation of shuddh (pure) ingredients, rice, and lentils, makes it ideal for periods of illness, detox, or ritual fasting.

I believe every region in India has its own version of khichdi:
- In Gujarat, it's often paired with kadhi (a yogurt-based curry).
- In Ayurveda, it is considered a sattvic dish, balancing the doshas and improving digestion.

Khichdi also has the unique status of being both everyday fare and ceremonial food, depending on how it's prepared. The turmeric not only imparts its signature golden hue but also acts as a healing agent, known for its anti-inflammatory and digestive properties. The choice of dal, my favorite, tuvar (pigeon peas) dal, also reflects regional preferences and seasonal needs. Combined with ghee, a source of healthy fat in Indian tradition, this dish becomes both nutrient-rich and easily digestible.

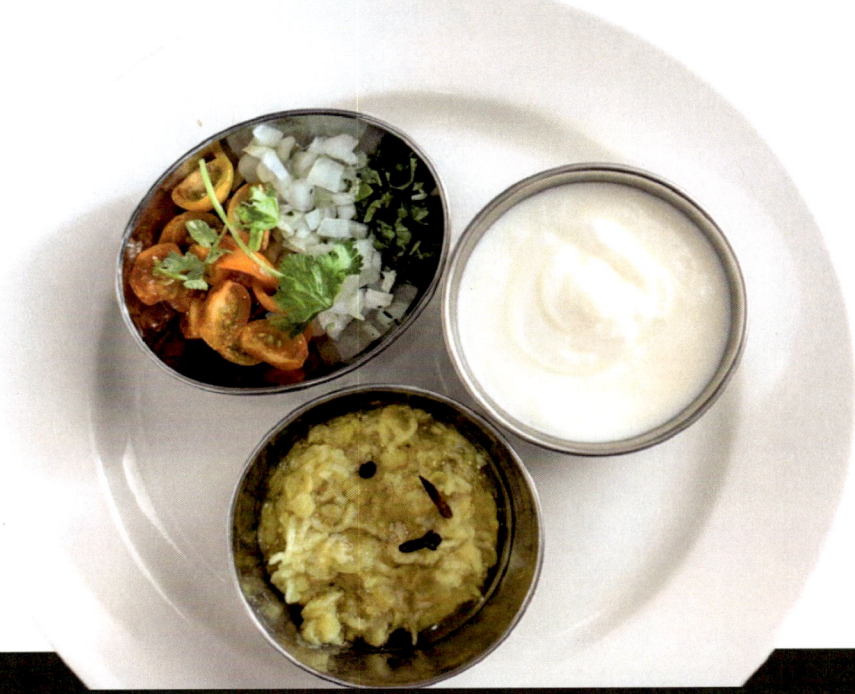

Khichdi is not just a meal; it is a comfort symbol of home, healing, and simplicity across the Indian subcontinent. With only a few pantry staples, rice, lentils, turmeric, and ghee, this dish comes together as a warm, golden porridge that generations have turned to for comfort, sustenance, and spiritual grounding.

Though humble in appearance, khichdi holds deep cultural meaning: it is often the first solid food fed to infants, a food for fasting and cleansing, and a dish deeply embedded in Ayurvedic tradition.

Ingredients

½ cup rice

½ cup tuvar dal (split pigeon peas)

4½ cups water

Salt to taste

¼ tsp turmeric

2 tbsp. oil or ghee

1 clove

1 cinnamon stick

Instructions

- **Soak the Grains**
1. Rinse and soak the rice and dal together for 30 minutes. Soaking is essential to ensure even cooking and better digestion.

- **Pressure Cook**
1. In a pressure cooker or Instant Pot, combine the soaked rice and dal with 4½ cups of water, turmeric, salt, clove, and cinnamon stick.
2. Seal the lid and pressure cook for 3 whistles (or for about 10 minutes on high pressure in an Instant Pot).
3. Let the pressure release naturally before opening.

- **Serve**
1. Once cooked, the khichdi should be soft and slightly mushy. Stir in a spoonful of ghee for richness.
2. If too dry, add a splash of hot water and mix. Serve hot.

Pro Tips and Customizations

- Use moong dal (yellow split mung beans) for a lighter, even more easily digestible version.
- Add vegetables like peas, carrots, or spinach to make it a full one-pot meal.
- For a deeper flavor, temper cumin seeds, ginger, or garlic in ghee and stir in after cooking.
- If reheating, add a splash of water to revive the creamy texture.

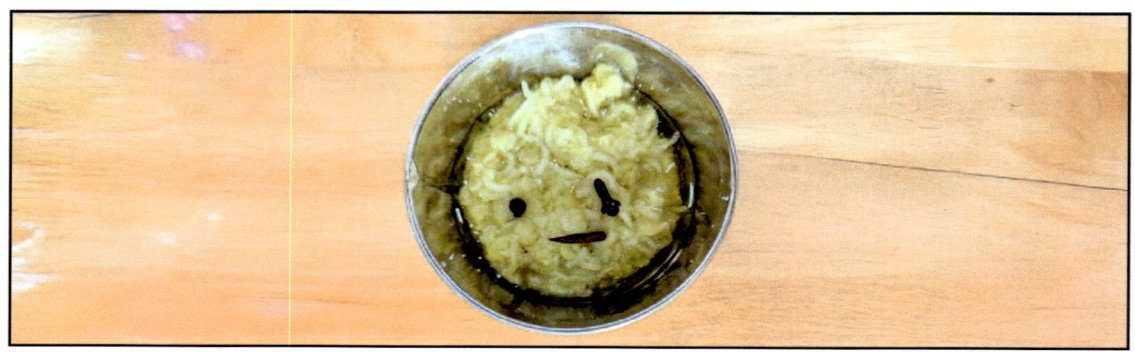

Whether you're under the weather or just in need of a little soul food, khichdi has a timeless way of wrapping you in warmth. Let it remind you of the power of simplicity, the heritage of home cooking, and the legacy of plant-based nourishment.

Bites

Peanut Brittle:

A SWEET LEGACY OF CRUNCH AND CRAFT

Sugar candies like brittle have an extensive history, dating back to ancient Persia and India, where early versions were made with honey and seeds or nuts. Peanut brittle, as known in the United States, likely emerged in the 19th century, becoming popular as corn syrup production expanded. In the American South, it's a common feature at fairs and holiday tables.

Peanuts themselves carry a global history; they originated in South America, were brought to Africa via Portuguese traders, and traveled to the U.S. with enslaved West Africans who adapted them into various dishes.

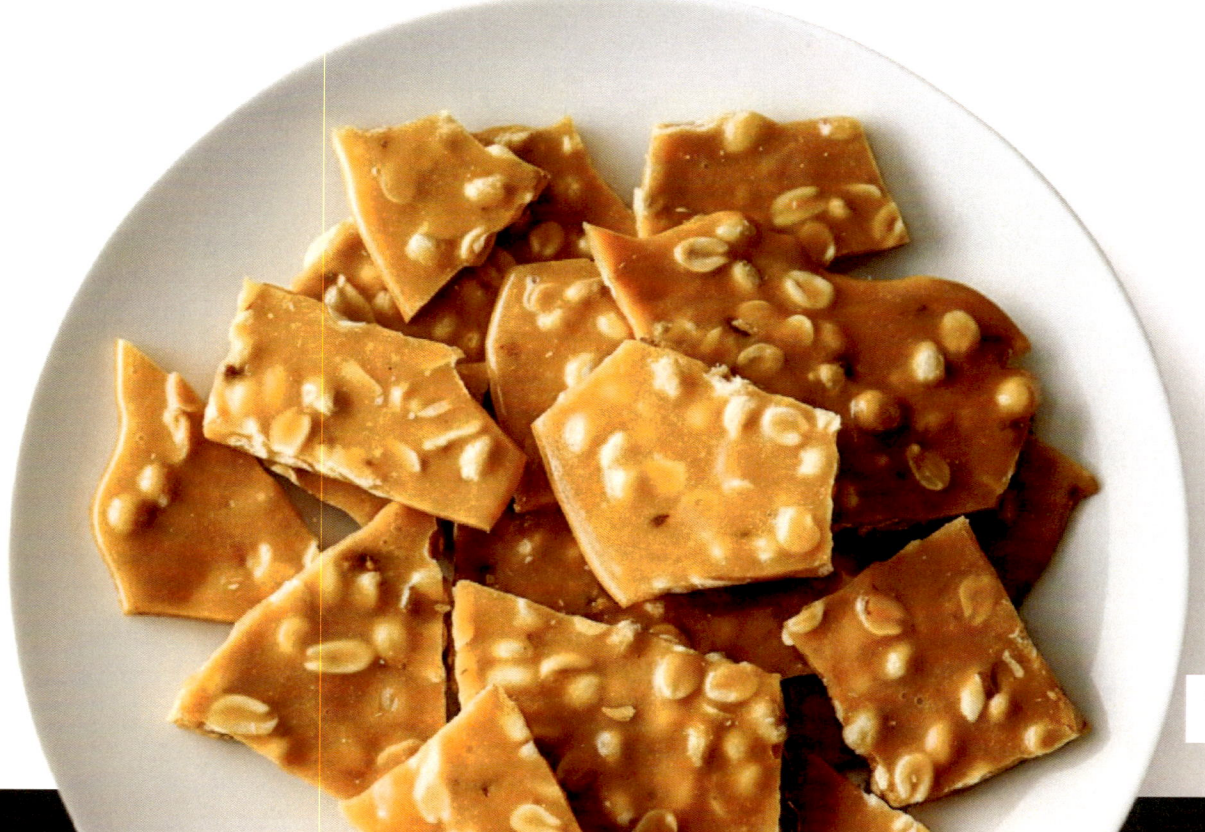

If you swap peanuts for sesame seeds, you're essentially making a sesame brittle, another similarly situated and equally popular sweet in India, especially during winter festivals like Makar Sankranti. Sesame, prized in Ayurvedic tradition for its warming properties, is believed to provide warmth, strength, and vitality, perfect for colder months.

Few confections bridge nostalgia and craftsmanship like peanut brittle. This golden, glossy candy is a beloved treat in many households, often passed down as a family recipe or handmade during festivals and holidays. Its satisfying crunch and caramelized, nutty flavor are matched only by its surprisingly ancient origins.

While this version uses peanuts, the brittle tradition spans continents. From Indian chikki made with jaggery and sesame, to Middle Eastern halva with pistachios, or Chinese huasheng tang, variations of nut-and-sugar candy speak to shared human cravings for sweetness and texture.

Ingredients

1 cup white sugar

½ cup light corn syrup

¼ tsp salt

¼ cup water

1 cup raw peanuts (or sesame seeds for variation)

2 tbsp. butter, softened

1 tsp baking soda

Instructions

- **Prep Your Workspace**

    Grease a large cookie sheet and set it aside. Candy hardens fast, so have everything ready before starting.

- **Cook the Syrup**

    In a heavy 2-quart saucepan, combine sugar, corn syrup, salt, and water. Bring to a boil over medium heat, stirring until the sugar dissolves.

- **Add the Nuts**

    Stir in peanuts and clip a candy thermometer to the side of the pot. Continue cooking, stirring frequently, until the temperature reaches 300°F (150°C), or until a drop hardens into brittle threads in cold water.

- **Finish and Pour**

    Remove from heat immediately. Stir in butter and baking soda, and it will foam and lighten the mixture. Quickly pour onto the cookie sheet. Use two forks to stretch the mixture into a thin rectangle (about 14x12 inches).

- **Cool and Snap**

    Let cool completely. Once hardened, break into pieces and store in an airtight container.

Pro Tips and Customizations

- Sesame Version: Use 1 cup of toasted white sesame seeds in place of peanuts. Stir them in after the syrup hits temperature. The result is thinner, more shattering, brittle, and great for gifting.

- Add a touch of vanilla extract for depth or a pinch of chili for heat.

- For a rustic version, replace white sugar with jaggery or coconut sugar.

- If using sesame, consider adding a sprinkle of sea salt or crushed cardamom on top before it cools.

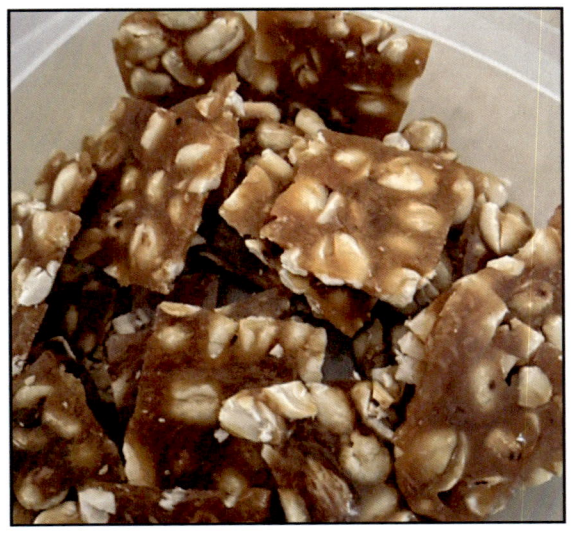

Whether you're using peanuts, sesame seeds, or something in between, brittle is a celebration of texture, tradition, and technique. It invites play and reminds us that even the simplest ingredients can transform into something extraordinary.

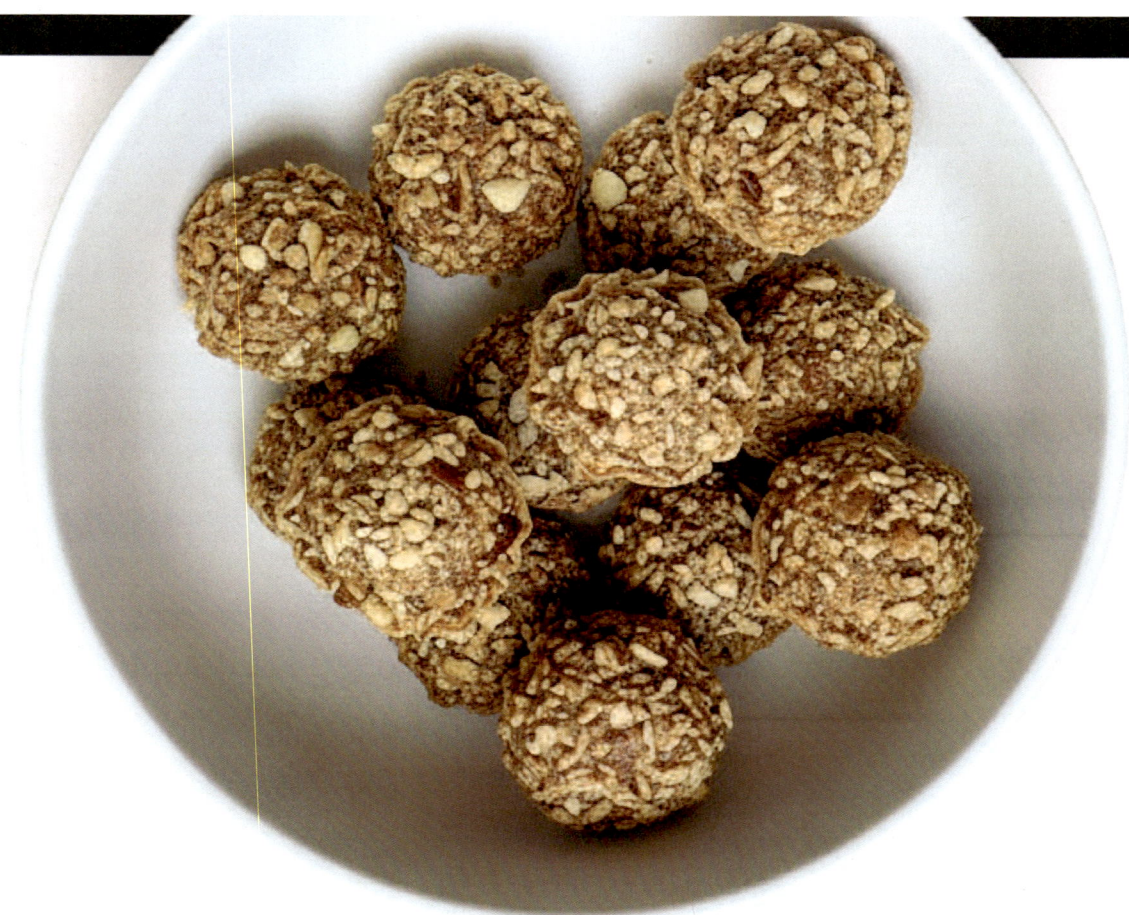

Chia Energy Bites:

ANCIENT SUPERFOODS IN A MODERN SNACK

Chia seeds were so vital to the Aztec civilization that they were often offered to the gods. Known for their ability to absorb water and form a gel-like consistency, they were consumed to increase stamina during long journeys or battles. The word "chia" itself comes from the Nahuatl word chian, meaning "oily", which also refers to their rich omega-3 content.

Coconut and honey each bring with them centuries of tradition. Honey, used in everything from Hippocratic medicine to Hindu rituals, represents both sustenance and sacredness. Coconut, meanwhile, is dubbed the "tree of life" in many cultures for its multitude of uses, from culinary to ceremonial.

By combining these ingredients into a single, convenient snack, this recipe reflects not just dietary mindfulness but also a deep connection to the food-ways of our ancestors.

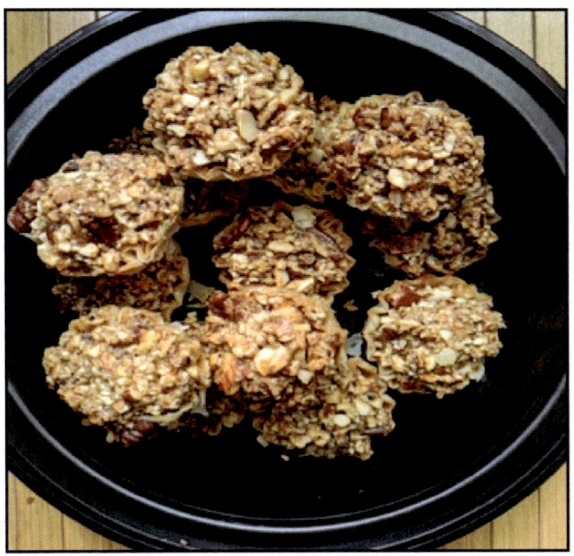

These chia energy bites are a no-bake snack that packs ancient wisdom into each bite. With ingredients like chia seeds, once prized by the Aztecs, and oats, which have nourished cultures across Europe for centuries, this recipe reminds us that modern health trends often have deeply traditional roots.

Perfect as a midday boost or a grab-and-go breakfast, these bites blend nutrient-dense whole foods in a way that feels effortless and satisfying. Best of all? No oven required.

Ingredients

- 1 cup rolled oats – A grain with deep roots in Northern Europe, oats are rich in fiber and known for their sustained energy release.

- 2 Tbsp. honey – Humanity's oldest natural sweetener, used medicinally and ritually from ancient Egypt to Vedic India.

- ½ tsp vanilla – A new world treasure cultivated by the Totonac people of Mexico long before it sweetened European confections.

- 2 Tbsp. whole chia seeds – Indigenous to Central America, chia was a dietary staple of the Aztecs, valued for endurance.

- ½ cup almond butter or peanut butter – Ground seed and nut pastes have long appeared in food cultures, from African groundnut stews to modern spreads.

- 2 Tbsp. shredded unsweetened coconut – Revered in South Asian and Pacific Island cultures for its versatility and nourishing fats.

Instructions

- Combine all ingredients in a large mixing bowl. Mix well until evenly blended.

- Using your hands or a spoon, roll into 16 bite-sized balls.

- Store in an airtight container in the refrigerator for up to one week.

> Optional: For extra texture, roll in crushed oats or coconut flakes before storing.

Pro Tips and Customizations

- Make it vegan: Use maple syrup or agave nectar instead of honey.

- Add-ins: Try flaxseed, chopped dried dates, or cacao nibs for variety.

- No nut butters? Try sun butter or tahini.

Think of these bites as tiny edible time capsules, offering sustenance from across civilizations in a form fit for a lunchbox or hiking trail.

Chinese Bhel:
STREET FOOD FUSION WITH GLOBAL ROOTS

Indo-Chinese cuisine emerged from Kolkata's Chinese immigrant community, particularly the Hakka people, who arrived in India in the 18th and 19th centuries. Over time, their techniques merged with Indian spices and ingredients, creating dishes like chili paneer, hakka noodles, manchurian, and, of course, Chinese bhel.

Chinese bhel likely developed in Mumbai's street food scene, taking the textural appeal of Indian chaats and combining it with spicy-sweet Chinese-style sauces. It reflects the post-colonial culinary fusion happening in urban India, where influences from China, Southeast Asia, and the West have been joyfully remixed.

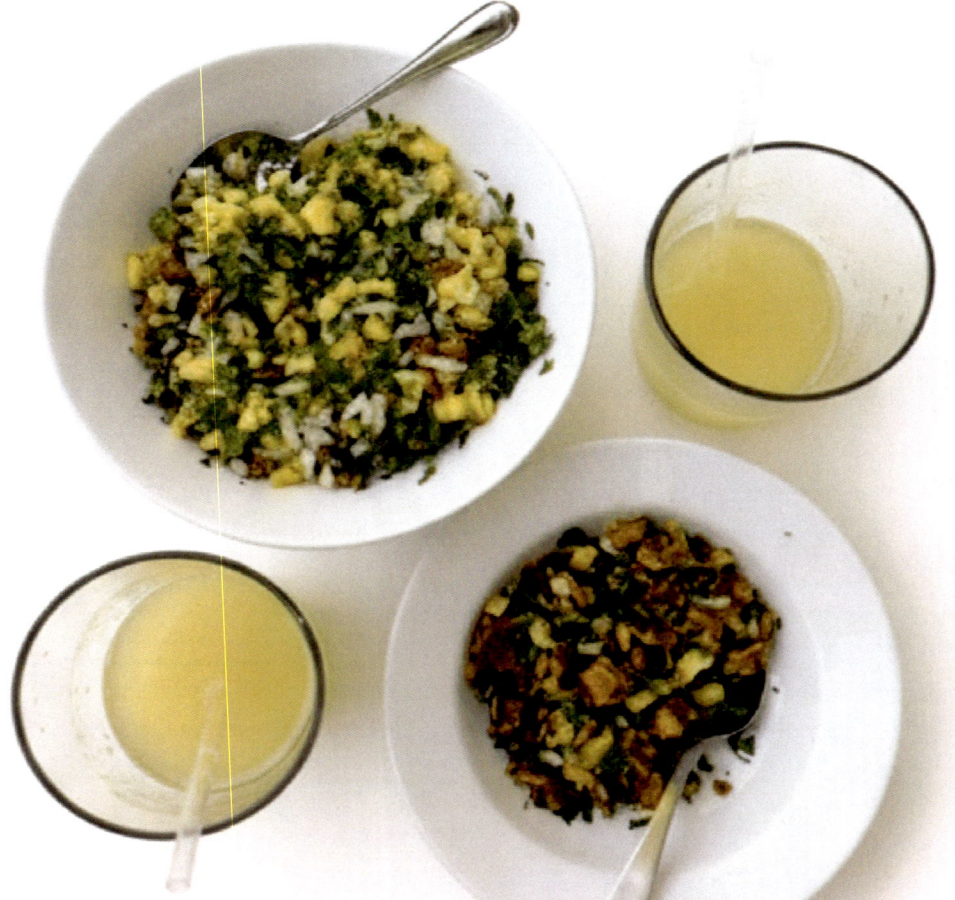

Interestingly, the inclusion of fried noodles mirrors how other popular Indian street foods are served, while ingredients like edamame or bell pepper show global adaptation and modern health trends.

Chinese bhel is a crispy, spicy, tangy, and wholly satisfying mashup born in the bustling lanes of Indian street food culture. It's not authentically Chinese, nor strictly Indian, but it's a joyful invention that perfectly captures India's long history of adapting global ingredients into something uniquely local. Also, this dish has a special place in my heart because of the family friend who has always been a presence in our family's biggest moments, whether joyful or troubling, who first introduced this fusion dish into our household!

Ingredients

FOR THE SAUCE (MAKES ENOUGH TO FILL A SMALL JAR):
½ cup oil
¼ cup finely chopped garlic
¼ cup finely chopped ginger
½ cup tomato purée
1½ cups red chili paste
Salt to taste
2 tbsp. sweet and sour sauce

2 tbsp. sriracha sauce
2 tbsp. soy sauce
2 tsp sugar
⅓ cup tomato ketchup (optional)
Optional: 1 tbsp. schezwan sauce for extra punch

FOR THE MIX
4 cups crunchy noodles (like thick sev, a crispy chickpea flour noodle, or other similar fried noodles)
½ cup chopped scallions
½ cup shredded cabbage
⅓ cup grated carrot
¼ cup thinly sliced bell pepper
½ cup edamame beans

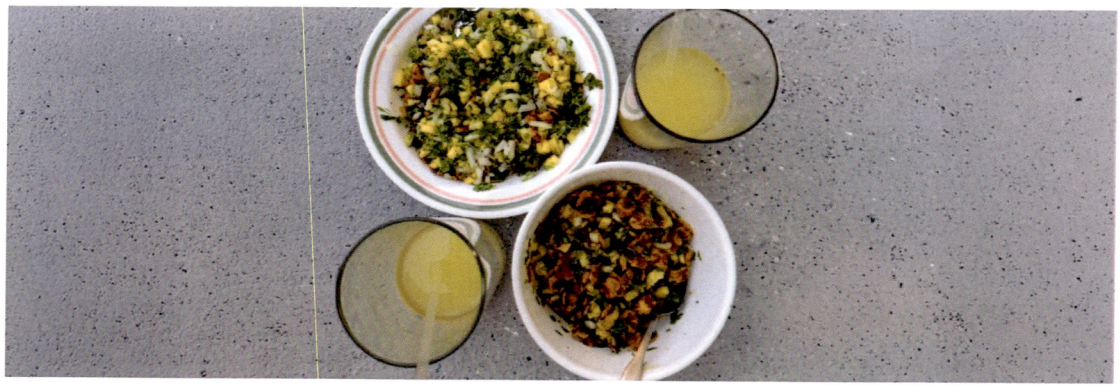

Optional additions: diced mango, chopped tomatoes, red onion, sprouted beans, because anything goes, just like traditional Indian bhel!

Instructions

- **Make the Sauce**

1. Heat oil in a pot until smoking. Add chopped garlic and ginger; sauté until fragrant.
2. Stir in the tomato purée and cook for a few minutes.
3. Add red chili paste and a splash of water. Simmer while stirring.
4. Add salt, sweet and sour sauce, sriracha, soy sauce, and sugar.
5. Optional: Add ketchup or schezwan sauce if using. Cook for 2–3 more minutes.
6. Let cool, then store in the fridge if making ahead.

- **Assemble the Chinese Bhel**

1. In a large bowl, combine the crunchy noodles, cabbage, carrots, bell peppers, edamame, and scallions.
2. Pour in the desired amount of sauce and toss well until evenly coated.
3. Serve immediately for max crunch!

Pro Tips and Customizations

- Add fruit: Ripe mango adds a sweet-tangy surprise.
- Protein boost: Add paneer cubes or tofu for a heartier version.
- Spice swap: If red chili paste is too intense, try chili garlic sauce instead.
- Texture tip: Toss just before serving because soggy noodles are a chaat faux pas.

Chinese bhel is a canvas for improvisation. Whether you're riffing on nostalgic chaat or serving it as a quirky party starter, this dish lets you travel through Mumbai, Kolkata, and Shanghai, all in one bite.

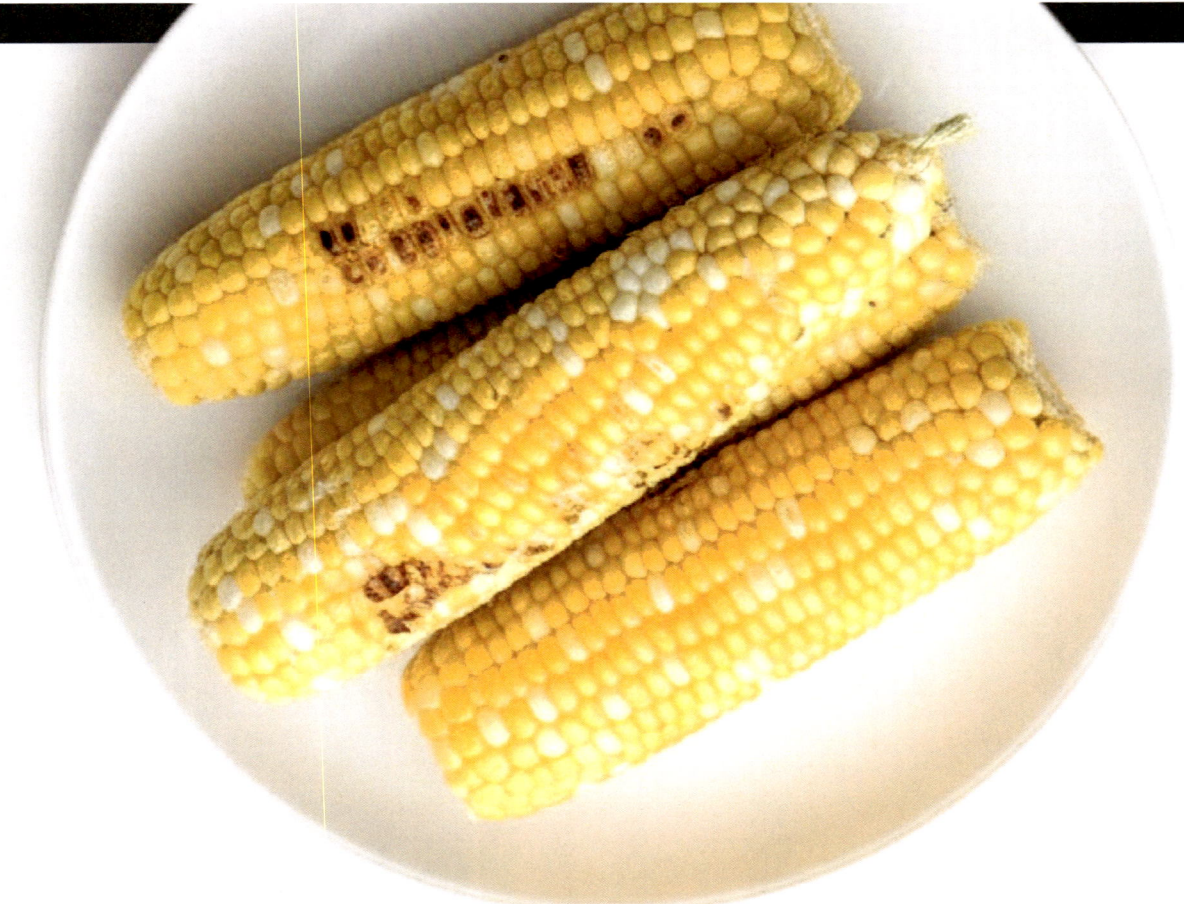

Esquites:

A TASTE OF MEXICAN STREET FOOD CULTURE

Corn, or maize, is not just the backbone of Mexican cuisine; it is part of the cultural heritage. Revered by indigenous civilizations such as the Aztecs and Mayans, corn was considered sacred and even used as currency. Over time, corn became a symbol of life and sustenance, its versatility reflected in dishes like tacos, tamales, and, of course, esquites (a popular Mexican street food made from roasted corn served with creamy, spicy toppings).

Esquites, also known as Mexican street corn in a cup, brings the flavors of a bustling Mexican street food vendor right to your home. This dish is a festive favorite in Mexico, where the smell of charred corn fills the air and vendors serve it with a combination of creamy, spicy, and tangy toppings. Esquites aren't just about food, but rather, it's about culture, connection, and enjoying the moment.

Whether served as a snack, appetizer, or side dish, esquites showcase the magical combination of corn, creamy mayonnaise, zesty lime, and bold chili flavors. This recipe brings the essence of Mexican street food to your kitchen.

Ingredients

- Vegetable oil – A neutral oil that helps achieve the perfect char on the corn kernels.

- Corn kernels – A staple ingredient in Mesoamerican cuisine, corn has been cultivated for thousands of years, revered by cultures like the Aztecs and Mayans.

- Salt – A universal seasoning with ancient roots, salt has been a key trading commodity since antiquity.

- Mayonnaise – While mayonnaise has European origins, its use in Mexican cuisine is a delicious twist on European dressings.

- Cotija cheese – This crumbly, salty cheese is often referred to as the "Parmesan of Mexico." Cotija is a symbol of Mexican dairy craftsmanship.

- Lime juice – Lime adds both tang and tradition, integral to Mexican flavor profiles.

- Chili powder – Chili peppers, a vital part of Mexican cuisine, have a long history dating back to indigenous cultures.

- Paprika – Derived from dried peppers, this spice brings depth and color to the dish.

- Scallions – A staple allium in many cuisines, scallions are used for both flavor and garnish.

- Cilantro – A herb deeply woven into Mexican food-ways, cilantro brings freshness and a pungent aroma to the dish.

- Garlic powder – Garlic has traveled the world from ancient Mediterranean and Middle Eastern kitchens, bringing warmth and savoriness to the mix.

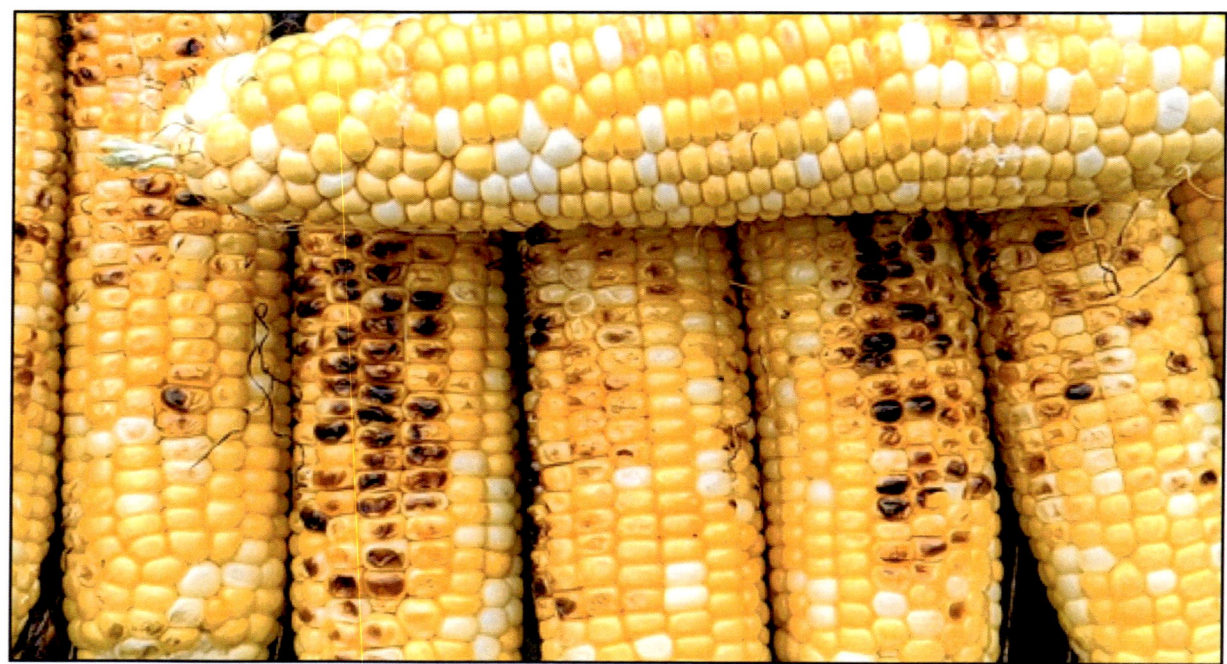

TIP: For added authenticity, Trader Joe's Everything but the Elote Seasoning is a great shortcut. It combines chili powder, cheese, and a bit of lime to mimic the traditional flavor profile of esquites.

Instructions

- **Char the Corn:**
1. Heat 1 tablespoon of vegetable oil in a large wok over high heat until it shimmers.
2. Add the corn kernels, season lightly with salt, and toss once or twice.
3. Cook until the corn is charred on one side, then toss and cook until charred on the second side. Continue tossing and charring until all sides are nicely roasted.

- **Mix the Ingredients:**
1. Transfer the charred corn into a bowl.
2. Add 1 tablespoon of mayonnaise, 1 ounce of crumbled cotija cheese, ½ tablespoon of lime juice, 1 teaspoon of chili powder, paprika, chopped scallions, cilantro, and garlic powder. Mix well.

- **Serve and Garnish:**
1. Serve warm, garnished with extra lime wedges and a sprinkle of chili powder for added spice.

Pro Tips and Customizations

- Use grilled corn: If you prefer a smoky flavor, grill your corn on the cob and cut it off after grilling to incorporate that extra char.
  Spice it up: For more heat, add a pinch of cayenne pepper or extra chili powder to your mix.
- Substitute: Use parmesan cheese if cotija is not available, or experiment with vegan mayo for a dairy-free version.

Esquites is the perfect party appetizer or side dish for your next barbecue or family gathering. The creamy, spicy, tangy, and crunchy combo makes it irresistible!

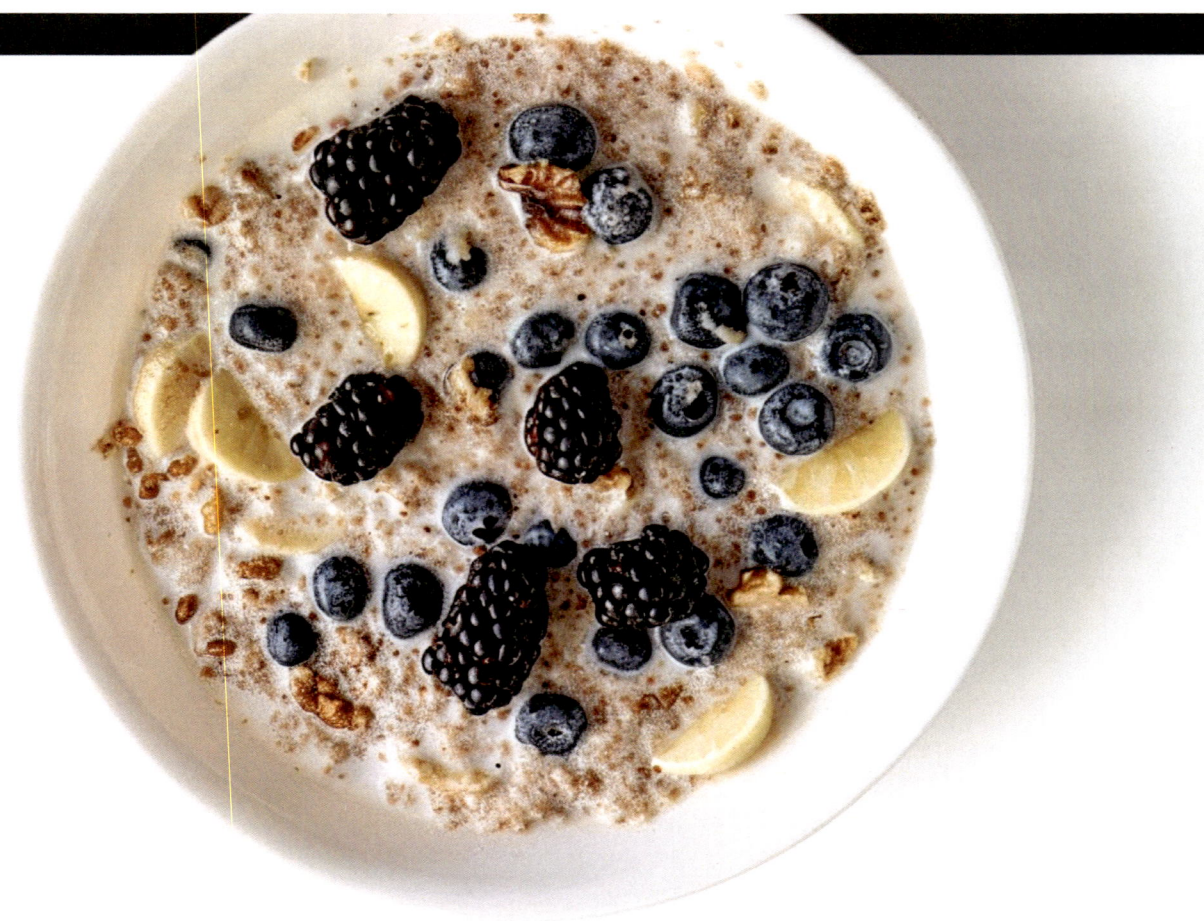

Overnight Blackberry Cinnamon Oats:

ANCIENT GRAINS MEET MODERN MORNINGS

Oats have been cultivated for over 2,000 years, originally as a weed in ancient wheat and barley fields. While often overshadowed by other grains, oats became a dietary cornerstone in Scotland and Northern Europe, prized for their hardiness and ability to grow in damp, cool climates. Porridge, made from oats, has long been associated with rustic nourishment and working-class roots.

Cinnamon, used here to add warmth, has a far more opulent origin story. Native to Sri Lanka and southern India, it was one of the first global commodities traded along the spice routes. In medieval Europe, it was more expensive than gold.

Blackberries, indigenous to North America and Europe, have long been foraged and celebrated in folk medicine for their antioxidant properties. Their presence in modern recipes like this represents a shift from wild harvest to everyday superfood.

Honey, a symbol of sweetness and health across cultures, from ancient Egypt to Ayurvedic India, has always had ritual and culinary significance, making even simple meals feel sacred.

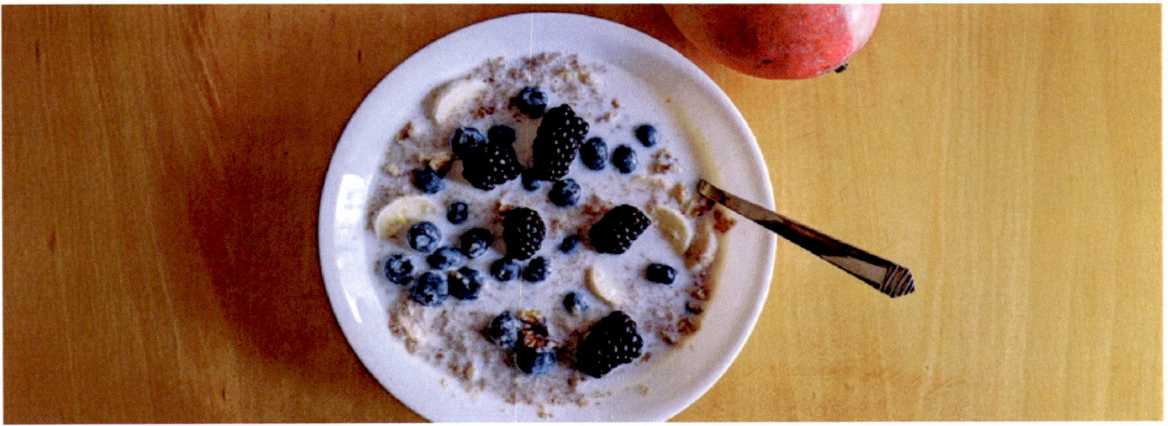

Quick, nourishing, and endlessly adaptable, overnight oats have become a staple of modern meal preparation with roots that go back centuries. This recipe pairs hearty old-fashioned oats with sweet-tart blackberries, warm cinnamon, and a hint of honey, creating a breakfast that feels both convenient and deeply comforting. Expect a mellow sweetness with a hint of warmth from cinnamon and bursts of berry brightness in every bite.

As food cultures evolve, old-world ingredients often find new expression. In this blend of the old and the new, every spoonful bridges rustic tradition with modern convenience. Here, oats, which were once a humble grain of the Scottish Highlands, combine with spices from Asia and berries native to North America, demonstrating how pantry staples can tell a global story.

Ingredients

1 cup old-fashioned oats

1½ cups fat-free milk (or dairy-free alternative)

½ tsp vanilla extract

⅛ tsp ground cinnamon (try a dash of nutmeg for additional warmth)

2 tsp honey (or substitute brown sugar)

1 cup fresh blackberries (or try blueberries or raspberries)

Pinch of salt

Instructions

- **Mix the Base**

  In a medium bowl, stir together oats, milk, vanilla, cinnamon, and a pinch of salt until well combined.

- **Divide and Top**

  Spoon the mixture into two resealable jars or containers. Top each with 1 tsp honey and ½ cup berries.

- **Chill Overnight**

  Seal and refrigerate for at least 6 hours or overnight.

- **Serve Warm**

  When ready to eat, uncover and microwave for 2–3 minutes until warmed through and tender. Stir and enjoy.

Pro Tips and Customizations

- Personally, I add 1 tbsp. chia seeds to the mix.
- Want more crunch? Top with toasted almonds or granola just before serving.
- Use plant-based milk to make it vegan.
- Stir in Greek yogurt for a protein boost.
- Try adding different fruits like bananas, apples, or mangoes!

This recipe shows how ancient ingredients can meet the needs of a fast-paced morning without losing their roots. Think about what berries, spices, or traditions you bring into your bowl!

Drinks

Mango Lassi:

A CREAMY, REFRESHING CLASSIC WITH A TROPICAL TWIST

Lassi is a traditional Indian drink with ancient roots, often made from yogurt blended with water and spices. Historically, lassi has been enjoyed not only as a refreshing drink but also for its cooling and digestive properties. Mango, native to South Asia, but now it is grown in almost all tropical climates, has long been cherished as the "king of fruits" for its sweetness and richness. Together, mango and yogurt form a beloved combination that represents the region's culinary heritage and connection to natural flavors.

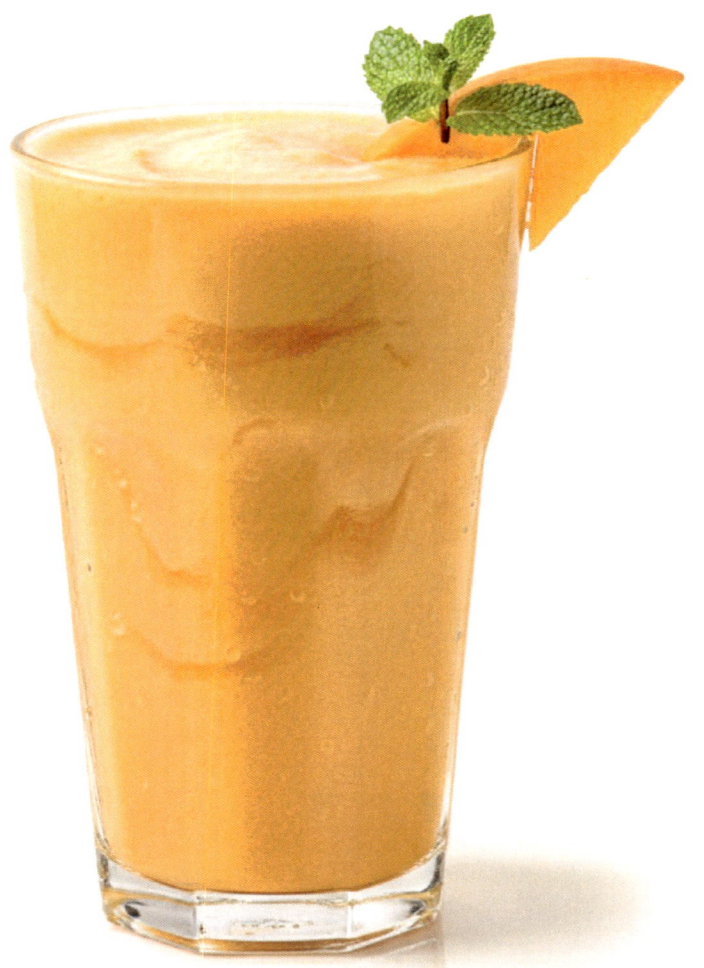

Mango lassi is a beloved, refreshing drink that perfectly balances creamy yogurt with the tropical sweetness of mangoes. Originating in India, lassi has been enjoyed for centuries as a cooling beverage, especially in the hot summer months. This version with mangoes adds a fruity twist to the traditional yogurt-based drink. Each sip brings me back to warm summer days spent with my family, enjoying homemade mango lassi as a treat to beat the heat. This simple recipe is a wonderful way to enjoy the rich flavors of ripe mango paired with a hint of cardamom for added depth.

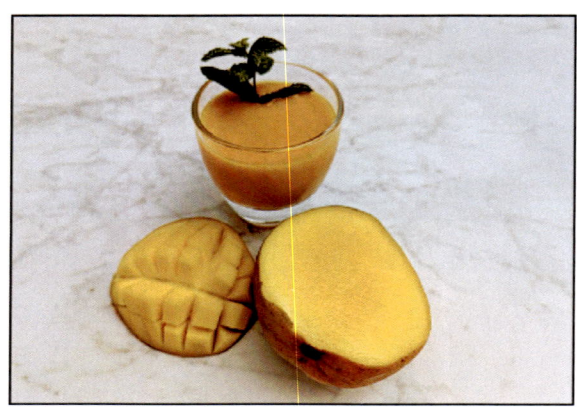

The great thing about this recipe is that you create the serving size based on the size and shape of your serving glasses. You can also add how many servings you want to make and adjust the total preparation time.

Ingredients

1 cup plain yogurt

½ cup milk

1 cup chopped very ripe mango (frozen or canned mango works too)

4 teaspoons honey or sugar (adjust to taste)

A dash of ground cardamom

Ice (optional, for a colder consistency)

Instructions

- Place mango, yogurt, milk, honey or sugar, and cardamom into a blender.

- Blend on high for 2 minutes until smooth and creamy.

- Pour into glasses and sprinkle with a tiny pinch of ground cardamom before serving.

- Optionally, blend in some ice or serve over ice for an extra-cool, milkshake-like consistency.

Note: Store any leftover lassi in the fridge for up to 24 hours.

Pro Tips and Customizations

- For a vegan option, use plant-based yogurt and milk alternatives, like coconut yogurt and almond milk.

- To make a thicker lassi, reduce the amount of milk or increase the yogurt.

- Adjust sweetness by adding more or less honey or sugar to suit your taste.

A quick and creamy mango lassi, with a hint of cardamom, is perfect for cooling down on a hot day or enjoying a taste of the tropics anytime! Whether you try it in the summer or try it in the winter, you'll surely sip on this exquisite taste!

Berry Smoothie:

A BLEND OF HEALTH AND HISTORY

There's something undeniably universal about the smoothie. This simple yet powerful drink ties modern nutritional science to ancient practices of food as medicine. My favorite berry smoothie is not just a refreshing start to the day; it's a blend of cultural and historical wisdom.

The blueberries in this recipe, known as nature's powerhouse of antioxidants, have roots in Indigenous North American diets, where they were used for nourishment and healing. Meanwhile, flaxseeds, once revered by ancient Egyptians, add fiber and omega-3s that support brain health and digestion. Even the simple banana, a staple of tropical agriculture for millennia, contributes its creamy texture and vitamin B6 to help recharge the body's detoxifying enzymes.

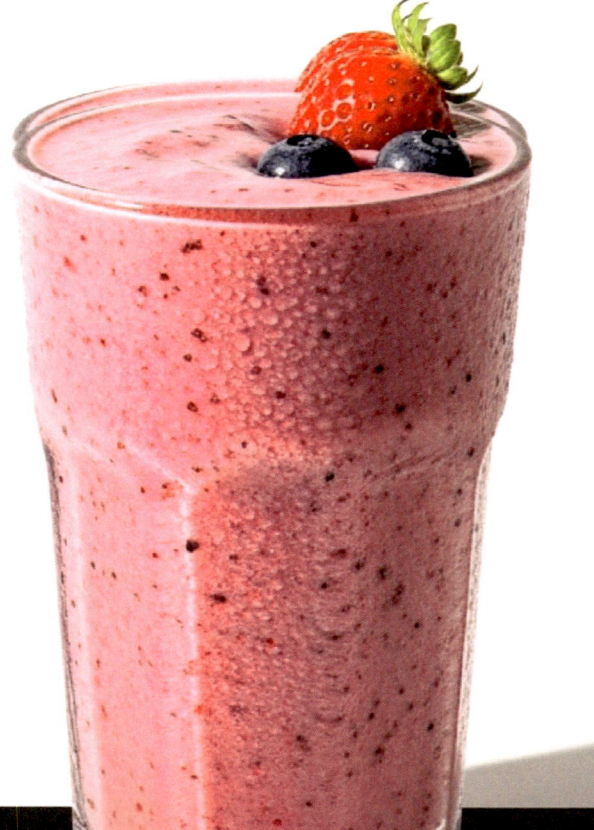

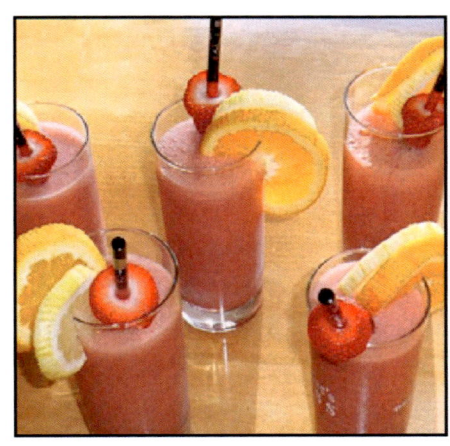

This smoothie goes beyond breakfast because it's a nourishing link to the past, blending modern wellness with timeless culinary traditions.

This berry smoothie is packed with antioxidants, fiber, and essential nutrients. Ready in under 5 minutes, it's the perfect way to start your day or recharge after school.

Ingredients

- 2 tablespoons protein powder – A modern addition, supporting muscle repair and overall wellness.

- 2 tablespoons ground flaxseeds – Cultivated since ancient Mesopotamian times, they're packed with omega-3s and fiber.

- 1/4 cup frozen berries – A colorful mix of antioxidants, historically used in Indigenous diets.

- 1/2 banana – A tropical fruit cultivated for over 7,000 years, adding sweetness and creaminess.

- 1 cup coconut water – The water of life in many tropical cultures, hydrating and rich in electrolytes.

Instructions

- Start with the liquid: Pour 1 cup of coconut water into your blender. Anthropological note: Coconut water has been a source of hydration for centuries in tropical regions, used both as sustenance and medicine.

- Add the dry ingredients: Add 2 tablespoons of protein powder and 2 tablespoons of ground flaxseeds. Note: Flaxseeds were considered sacred by ancient civilizations, often used for medicinal purposes and rituals.

- Add the fruit: Toss in 1/4 cup of frozen berries and 1/2 banana. Did you know? Berries have been a dietary staple for Native Americans, who dried them to preserve their nutrients for winter.

- Blend until smooth: Start on low speed and gradually increase for a velvety consistency. Pro Tip: Always add your ingredients in this order—liquid, powder, solids—for the smoothest blend.

- Save the rest: Freeze the other half of the banana for tomorrow's smoothie or a quick snack.

Pro Tips and Customizations

- For an added protein boost, try Greek yogurt instead of protein powder.

- Substitute chia seeds for flaxseeds; they've been cultivated by the Aztecs since 3500 BCE.

- Use almond milk instead of coconut water for a creamier texture and a reflection of Mediterranean culinary traditions.

- Decorate your cup with fruit (strawberries and oranges)!

I hope this berry smoothie becomes a staple in your morning routine, just as it has in mine. Cheers to starting your day with a delicious connection to the past and a boost for the

Epilogue

As a kid, dinner was like a hostage negotiation, and the broccoli always won. While my friends chased cupcakes and cronuts, I was just trying to swallow a spoonful of yogurt without flinching. I grew up seeing meals not as moments of joy, but as hurdles to clear. That daily struggle, though, laid the groundwork for transformation. I've been swept up in the age of hyperflavor, only for me, it's deeply personal.

What once felt like a burden has become a passion. As a self-taught teenage chef, I was determined to create flavors I actually wanted to eat. Now I find joy in bold, layered ingredients: golden saffron linguine with its floral aroma; pistachio broccoli pesto with its earthy complexity; cinnamon-infused French toast stuffed with strawberries, a dish that tastes like a hug on a plate.

These are not just recipes; they are milestones in my journey from disdain to creativity. Notice how our collective taste buds are evolving and awakening as we try new ingredients and develop new flavors. Cooking is a way to reclaim curiosity, joy, and identity through ingredients that once may have felt out of reach. We are not chasing a hype or fad; we are chasing possibility. And these days, I'm hungry, not disheartened. In fact, the broccoli doesn't win anymore. I do.

Acknowledgements

First up, a huge thank-you to Masi, my mom's younger sister, my partner in late-night snack crimes and kitchen chaos. Whether we were experimenting with something new or just making a delicious mess, you always made it fun (and somehow tasty). You've earned honorary degrees in both midnight munchies and culinary creativity.

Kush, thank you for the endless stories at the dinner table that made meals feel more like a comedy show (with intermissions for chewing). Your loyalty to a predictable menu has, on occasion, made me look like a daring foodie by comparison. Much appreciated.

Dad, thank you for being the ultimate partner when it comes to buying groceries, not only for always driving and paying, but also for encouraging me to try new things. Our adventures started when we enjoyed the simple pleasures like watching the train go around the tracks at Wegmans in Burlington, MA, before picking up fun ingredients like fat-free crumbled feta cheese and low-fat kefir! Here's to many more food shopping adventures.

Ritaba, thank you for always being in the kitchen, cooking with love and intention. Your food is comfort, tradition, and pure magic rolled into every bite.

Dada, thank you for being the family's recipe inventor. Your creative dishes somehow always work out, and your kitchen experiments are the delicious proof that good food starts with curiosity.

Pakaba and Nirudada, thanks for cooking the same foods when we visit. It has become a routine expectation, which is something I can count on.

Kaka, Kaki, Rahi, and Baby Kai, I feel like you love me just as I am and make it fun for me to just be me. We laugh about anything when we are together, whether it be serving food at parties, looking through a snack-filled pantry, or searching for both familiar favorites and new ingredients on a menu at a new restaurant.

Masa, my masi's husband, thank you for your dedication to culinary precision. Only you would watch ten YouTube videos to figure out how to make the "perfect" version of a dish, even if it's just roasted potatoes. Your commitment to the craft is inspiring (and very tasty).

To my feeding therapists, Ellen Gellineau and Arden Hill, you helped me feel brave and capable in ways that go far beyond the table. Thank you for your care and patience. To my amazing nutritionists, Katie, Anne, Fran, Heidi, and Dominica, thank you for keeping things balanced (even when I wasn't).

And shout-out to the instructors who showed me that cooking could be fun and delicious: the folks at Cozy Meals, Kids Cooking Green, Kid's Test Kitchen, and to Ming Tsai, whose cookbook and stories helped me see food as something joyful, personal, and powerful.

Also, a note to my extended family members, some of you may not know it, and others I may not have told in-person, but I have sincerely found joy in food every time we have sat around a table together, from the food we ate to the stories we shared.

And finally, Mom. The MVP. The kitchen wizard. The one-woman catering service. Thank you for always making sure there's something for me to eat at all times, including the times I did not even realize I was hungry. Even when you are running on an empty fuel tank, you manage to whip up magic. Your dedication to keeping me (and my brother) fed, with love, variety, and snacks in between, deserves a lifetime achievement award.

About the Author

Arjun Patel has been passionate about food for as long as he can remember. As a little kid, he is often remembered as the one who told friends and teachers that he wanted to be a chef or a food scientist, even asking for multiple cooking-related birthday parties growing up. His love for cooking and helping others enjoy food began at age two, when he started a 'failure to thrive' five-year journey through feeding therapy. There, he learned not just to eat, but to truly connect with food, its flavors, textures, and the stories it tells.

Born in Boston and raised in Lexington, Massachusetts, Arjun continues to explore food in creative and joyful ways. When he's not in the kitchen, he enjoys bird watching, sewing, reading books, and playing board games with family and friends.

Through his recipes and his story, Arjun hopes to inspire other kids to be curious about food, try new things, and find their own joy in the kitchen, one bite at a time.

www.ingramcontent.com/pod-product-compliance
Lightning Source LLC
Chambersburg PA
CBRC091503220426
43661CB00021B/1306